# GREEN
# BARBARIANS

How to Live Bravely on Your Home Planet

ELLEN SANDBECK

Scribner

NEW YORK   LONDON   TORONTO   SYDNEY

Scribner
A Division of Simon & Schuster, Inc.
1230 Avenue of the Americas
New York, NY 10020

First Scribner trade paperback edition January 2010

SCRIBNER and design are registered trademarks of The Gale Group, Inc., used under license by Simon & Schuster, Inc., the publisher of this work.

For information about special discounts for bulk purchases, please contact Simon & Schuster Special Sales at 1-866-506-1949 or business@simonandschuster.com.

The Simon & Schuster Speakers Bureau can bring authors to your live event. For more information or to book an event contact the Simon & Schuster Speakers Bureau at 1-866-248-3049 or visit our website at www.simonspeakers.com.

Manufactured in the United States of America

2   4   6   8   10   9   7   5   3   1

Library of Congress Control Number: 2009021069

ISBN 978-1-4165-7182-7
ISBN 978-1-4165-7690-7 (ebook)

This book is dedicated to everyone who knows that
"because we say so" is not an answer.

# Contents

Preface · xi

Introduction: Bravery · 1

One: The Barbarian Body · 27

Two: At the Barbarian's Table · 62

Three: The Barbarian's Kitchen · 129

Four: The Barbarian Bathroom · 151

Five: Barbarian Laundry · 166

Six: Barbarically Healthy · 183

Seven: Barbarian Pets · 211

Eight: Little Barbarians · 218

In Conclusion · 240

Acknowledgments · 245

Bibliography · 247

Index · 261

# GREEN
## BARBARIANS

# Preface

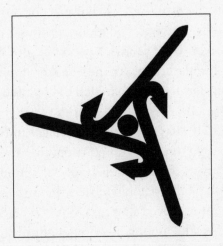

I got the idea for this book as my husband and I were eating a picnic lunch in front of a bonfire in our back four. (We own five acres. A back forty is beyond our capabilities.) My husband, who is more domestic than I, brought a tray loaded with a lovely post-Thanksgiving feast: hot spiced apple cider in a jar; capicola ham; smoked cheese; homemade bread; goat cheese; apples; and pumpkin pie. I was happily contemplating the prospect of enhancing my garden beds with charcoal dust from the soon-to-be-quenched fire, and wondering whether I should wipe the capicola grease on my husband's pants, since he had forgotten to bring out napkins, and his pants were dirtier than mine, when it occurred to me that a barbarian would wipe her hands on her slice of bread. So I did, and as I did, I realized that it might be time to resurrect the concepts of bread-napkins, trenchers, and other premodern conveniences. After much labor, and many more than nine months later, this book was born. It is filled with domestic strategies both ancient and modern—many delicious, all amusing—that I hope will improve the lives of ecologically minded people, and perhaps serve as a guide to the more feral side of life.

Those who walk the wilder, less-trodden path have always served as scouts for the rest of us. These venturesome souls are the explorers, the discoverers, the early adopters who help blaze the trails that will eventually take the rest of us where we need to go. Human survival has always depended upon intrepid individuals who cannot wait to discover what is just around the bend, on the other side of the river, or beyond the hills. They call to us from cliff tops, treetops, and mountaintops, saying, "Look! We've just found a new food or water source, a good place to make camp, or tool-making material." Nowadays, many of these seekers wave to us from bicycles and skateboards, from cars that belch french fry–scented exhaust, from thrift stores and rooftop gardens, even from Dumpsters.

Almost immediately after the atrocious attacks in September 2001, the Powers That Be strongly urged us to go shopping; they informed us that our economy rested upon the backs of shoppers, without whom our entire culture would collapse. This may have been the first time in recorded history that a government deployed shoppers to protect a country from attack. Now perhaps the renegades among us who delight in thumbing their noses at (and sometimes even sticking their thumbs into the eyes of) the agro-pharmo-military-industrial complex may reasonably be considered members of a new tribe of barbarians: the Green Barbarians.

The classical Greek and Latin definitions of barbarian simply meant one who was not of the dominant culture, and who was therefore considered strange or bizarre. Green Barbarians are those who define themselves by what they do and what they create, what they save and what they preserve, rather than by what they buy and what they consume. Thus the horde of Green Barbarians marches firmly upstream, against the flow of consumerist propaganda.

Taking the free advice Big Business so generously provides has enticed us into a trap baited with toxic food, drink, and playthings. Maybe it's time to learn from the wild ones who are searching for a way out of the trap. Advances in science and technology have given us ways to live longer, healthier lives, with a greatly reduced incidence (in the First World) of infectious diseases caused by poor sanitation. However, we may have made a mistake when we threw the barbarian out with his dirty bathwater. That bathwater probably contained everything from beneficial insects, to immunity-building bacteria, to inoculating dirt that could have protected us from asthma, allergies, and autoimmune disorders. In some ways, our hypersanitized, consumer-product-driven culture has made us sick. Ancient barbarians may have lived short, brutal lives, but it is highly unlikely that they suffered from asthma, hay fever, diabetes, or ulcerative colitis. Nor were they beautifying themselves or their surroundings with products so full of hormones that they polluted the waters and forced male fish to fully explore their feminine side.

If you've lain awake nights anxious, worrying about how clean—or unclean—your house is, this book is for you. If you've ever wondered "Are these leftovers safe?," this book is definitely for you; if you would like to spend less time cleaning your house and more time doing things that you *really* enjoy, this book will show you the shortcuts. If your dog is having inexplicable coughing fits that last most of the day, this book is for you. (Note: The dog may be reacting to that plug-in "air freshener." Unplug it and throw it away.)

If your idea of a ripsnorting good time is to don heavy clothing, a hard hat, and safety goggles, and then run at high speed through pitch-black woods until you fall over, this book is really for you! If you pride yourself on your ability to eat bizarre foods; if your loyal gym socks stand up by themselves in a corner of your room until you need them again; if you only clean before company comes, and sometimes not even then, this book is for you. If you've ever tried to clean the mineral deposits out of your toilet bowl with a power grinder, this book is for you. If your cat refuses to enter your bathroom in order to use its litter box, this book is for you. If you are already a barbarian, this book will help you become a Green Barbarian. (Note to self: Would a paste of woad and turmeric turn the skin green? Investigate.)

Our home planet is, after all, planet Earth, not planet Just-cleaned-deodorized-disinfected-shined-bleached-and-polished. Life here can be a bit scary. It is frequently dirty, grimy, and gritty, and it is, and always has been, bacteria-laden. These are not sufficient reasons for letting the advertisers scare us into emptying our pockets and poisoning ourselves. Use what you have at hand in new and innovative ways. Take stock of what you have in abundance. Frustrate and thwart the powers that be. Use your mind, hands, and heart to make a better life for yourself and for those you love.

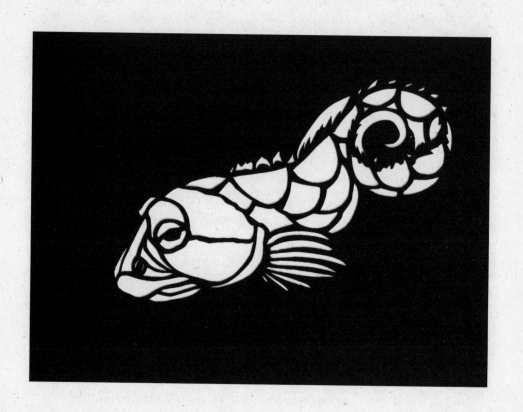

# Bravery

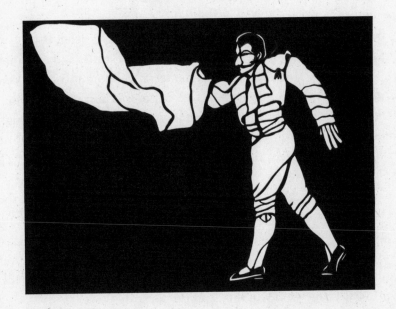

To believe yourself brave is to be brave; it is the one only essential thing.

—Mark Twain, *Personal Recollections of Joan of Arc*

When I began doing the research for this book, I thought I had a fairly good idea of what I would find. I could not have been more mistaken. I thought I understood that Big Business is only interested in money, not in improving their customers' lives, but when I really began digging, I was deeply shocked by the astounding depth, breadth, and density of Big Business's indifference not only to their customers' well-being, but also to the common good and the survival of our biosphere. I hunted down leads for days, trying to make connections between maternal diet and birth defects, and was successful in making these connections more often than I had any right to expect. I was nauseated for a week while researching and writing about the health effects of some hair care products. I read scientific papers that made my hair stand on end, and my hair is thick, heavy, and a foot and a half long. I discovered the truth, and the truth is that Big Business does not give a damn about you or your family, and it never has.

Big Business does not care whether you are alive or dead, it just wants your money, and the main tool it uses to empty your wallet is fear. You may think you are buying that face cream, shampoo, deodorant, or fancy purse because it will make you more attractive and more desirable, but the real message underlying the advertising is that if you are not beautiful enough, or don't smell good enough, you will be lonely. You may think you are buying that fabric softener, bleach, dish liquid, air freshener, floor wax, or "weed-and-feed" product because you love your family and want your home to be pleasant and attractive, but the advertisers' underlying message is that if you don't keep your home up, your neighbors will disapprove, and you and your entire family will be lonely outcasts. You may think you are buying that antibacterial aerosol air freshener because you want to do the best thing for your family, but the underlying message is really that if you don't kill all the bacteria in your home, you will die.

Much modern advertising is pure fear-mongering. You can save your money and your health by educating yourself so you can distinguish between a real threat and an advertising ploy, and then you can act accordingly. Whenever someone tells you that you need to be afraid of something, and that person conveniently happens to sell the perfect product to defuse that threat, you can never go wrong by asking yourself whether the threat is real or whether it is just a sales pitch. Advertising has made us fearful, and fear is dangerous. I hope this book will help people pry themselves away from harmful products they don't need and the environment can't afford. I also hope readers will take away the message that people who are willing to dig deeply and in the right places can unearth information that can dramatically change their outlook.

I do not consider myself a particularly brave person, and I am generally quite sanguine when confronted by utter harmlessness. But I do try to keep myself well informed so I can be appropriately cautious when faced with real danger. This attitude obviously leaves me quite far from the realm of heroism, but I lead a fairly quiet life that rarely necessitates actual bravery.

I am not generally afraid of spiders (spider-bite fatalities in the United States in 1997: zero) nor am I frightened of most snakes (snakebite fatalities in the United States over a recent twenty-year period: 97). Even the West Nile virus does not particularly alarm me (161 deaths in the United States in 2006). During the panicky season of 2002–2003, I was quite optimistic about my chances of surviving SARS (severe acute respiratory syndrome), which killed 801 people worldwide, and no one in the United States. And I'm usually not worried about shark attacks. Shark-bite fatalities in the United States average one per year or fewer, though in Minnesota, where I do most of my swimming, the annual number of shark attacks is generally zero. (Although in August 2004, an eleven-year-old boy who was wading in Island Lake needed eleven stitches after he was bitten by either a muskellunge or a northern pike.)

Though I am brave in the presence of spiders, I have a healthy fear of handguns (gun fatalities in the United States in 1998: 30,088). I am terrified by incapacitated drivers (drunk driving fatalities in the United States in 2004: 16,694) and by drivers who are talking on the phone, eating, smoking, reading the newspaper, drinking coffee, and shaving and/or applying makeup while driving. (According to the National Highway Traffic Safety Institute and the Virginia Tech Transportation Institute, nearly 80 percent of crashes and 65 percent of near-misses involve drivers who were distracted within three seconds of the event.) And since we moved to our rural home in 2000, I have begun to flinch at the sight of an oncoming gravel truck. We have had four windshields cracked by projectiles ejected from uncovered gravel trucks; I reckon that every time we head toward town, we have approximately a 1 in 750 chance of a gravel strike.

But what really frightens me, in a lasting and permanent way, is the ongoing degradation, destruction, and poisoning of our environment. This fear is, unfortunately, rather all-encompassing, since environmental degradation, like greed, easily crosses geographical boundaries and political barriers. A study released by the World Health Organization in October

2006 estimates that air pollution causes the premature deaths of two million people every year. More than half of these victims are poor and live in developing countries, and up to 750,000 of those victims were Chinese. The Chinese government unsuccessfully attempted to suppress this dismal statistic by pressuring the World Bank to delete the mortality numbers from the formal draft of the 2007 report "Cost of Pollution in China." As Shakespeare wrote, "in the end, truth will out."

Before we climb onto our high horse to look down upon China's pitifully polluted soil, water, and air, we should ask ourselves whose filthy lucre finances that pollution. It turns out that more than $232.5 billion worth of China's environmentally costly goods were exported to the United States so that Americans could buy dirt cheap whaddyacallems. Unfortunately, cheap is not simply "1 a: purchasable below the going price or the real value," it is also "3 a: of inferior quality or worth . . . b: contemptible because of lack of any fine, lofty, or redeeming qualities" (*Webster's Collegiate Dictionary*, 11th Edition).

In 1977, the Consumer Product Safety Commission (CPSC) issued a final ban on lead-containing paint on toys and furniture in order to reduce the risk of lead poisoning in children. Between 1977 and the end of the twentieth century, there were a total of six recalls of toys due to excessive lead content. The largest was in 1994, when 996,547 individual boxes of Chinese-made coloring crayons plus 430 cases of the same types of crayons were recalled. The pace increased in 2003, when 1.4 million lead-based children's necklaces from India were recalled. In 2005, several thousand lead-based children's bracelets from China were recalled. In 2006, there were 5 lead-induced recalls of toys—4 of the recalls were of Chinese-made toys, and 1 was of toys from Hong Kong. So far, the biggest year for recalls of toxic children's toys was 2007—by November, more than 5 million toys had been recalled because they contained enough lead to harm or kill children who sucked on or swallowed them.

"There is no safe dose of lead."
—David Jacobs, former director, Office of Healthy Homes
and Lead Hazard Control of the U.S. Department
of Housing and Urban Development

Recent studies suggest that children's IQs drop six points even when their blood-lead levels are well below the levels the CPSC considers too high. And adults should not be too complacent about their own risks from lead: Some studies suggest that a failing memory may not be a normal sign of aging, but rather a sign that one has ingested too much lead, and a study published by the American Heart Association in 2006 links high lead levels to an increased risk of stroke.

## CREATIVE CONTAMINATION

The much-heralded Aqua Dots toy, one of the leading contenders for "gotta have it" toy of the 2007 Christmas season, was recalled in November 2007 because children who swallowed the little beads had fallen into comas. When swallowed, the water-soluble glue in the beads metabolized into gamma-hydroxybutyrate (GHB), the "date rape" drug. (And who could possibly have predicted that children might swallow small, brightly colored beads?) An overdose of GHB can cause seizures, coma, or death. The Aqua Dots factory is located in Shenzhen, in the province of Guangdong in China. GHB's precursor chemical, gamma-butyrolactone (GBL), is a solvent that is used in floor-cleaning products, paints, metal-etching solutions, batteries, nail polish, pesticides, and superglue removers. The Chinese manufacturer had substituted the toxic but cheap solvent for a much more expensive water-soluble glue that was in the toy's original specifications.

## WHAT GOES AROUND COMES AROUND

According to the U.S. State Department's report on China, "respiratory and heart diseases related to air pollution are the leading cause of death in China," and "every day approximately 300 million residents drink contaminated water."

China is the ultimate destination of 70 percent of the computers, TVs, cell phones, and other electronic waste (e-waste) that is recycled in the

United States. A study led by Ming H. Wong tested the dioxin levels at an e-waste recycling site in China, and found that they were twenty-five times higher than the World Health Organization's tolerable daily limit for adults. (Since dioxins are produced when plastics and other chlorine-containing compounds are burned, the contamination at this site was probably the result of burning the plastic insulation and plastic casings off of wires and electronics.) Exposure to dioxins disrupts the endocrine system; impairs the immune system; interferes with reproduction; reduces men's testosterone levels and decreases sperm production; causes birth defects such as spina bifida; causes developmental disabilities; increases the risk of cancer, heart disease, and diabetes; and increases the risk of childhood leukemia.

But eventually what goes around comes around. Chinese air pollution does not obediently stay put over China; instead, it goes wandering all over the planet, and eventually darkens the skies over the United States, precipitating out in the form of mercury-contaminated acid rain. And products produced in China wander all over the world as well.

Jeffrey Weidenhamer, a chemistry professor at Ashland University in Ohio, studied the cheap, lead-based Chinese jewelry that has been recalled in the past few years in the United States, and found that some of these baubles were made of mixtures of lead, copper, and tin that closely matched the metal mixtures found in the solder and circuit boards in computers and other electronics. Other cheap jewelry that Professor Weidenhamer tested was made of metal that strongly resembled the mixture of lead and antimony found in lead batteries. Obviously, banishing our dangerous trash to the other side of the planet is no guarantee that our poisons will not come back to haunt us. We need to insist that manufacturers produce goods that are safe and nontoxic at every stage of their lives, including after they have ceased to function; and we need to insist that all imported goods be subjected to meaningful, comprehensive safety inspections before they are allowed into the country. There is no such thing as "away."

There is no such thing as a free lunch, and generally there is no such thing as a cheap and healthy one either. Cheap is usually cheap for a reason. Is it really so surprising that Chinese manufacturers do not care about the health of little American children? Over the past several years,

American consumers have made it abundantly clear that the lowest possible price is of the utmost importance. The Chinese factories are just giving us what we want. To paraphrase Pogo, "We have the met the polluter, and he is us."

## AMERICA'S NATIONAL SPORT

Why are we so hell-bent on buying cheap stuff? I think some of it has to do with America's *real* national sport: competitive shopping. Often when I bought things for our children when they were small, I would casually mention it to an acquaintance, who would then launch into a song-and-dance number: "Oh, I can't believe you bought that for that much! I just checked out all the stores and bought one for half that!" That competitive shopper had probably spent many hours and wasted a lot of gasoline in order to save five dollars. I would much rather spend a little more money and far less time and energy to get what I need. Better yet, I'd rather save up and buy something that is well made by workers who are paid a living wage by an industry that produces as little pollution as possible.

My own career as a competitive shopper ended before it had even begun: When I was a teenager, I went to an après-Noël sale at a ritzy department store in San Francisco with my mother. I was casually approaching a sales table, and must have gotten too close to something that a little old lady coveted, because she hit me over the head with her handbag. There are no material goods I want that desperately. I can wait.

A *Harper's* magazine survey conducted in October 2001 found that 52 percent of American women prefer shopping to sex; 93 percent of men prefer sex.

The lust for more and cheaper stuff endangers both human and environmental health. But because consumerism/materialism has crept very close to the space often occupied by religion and patriotism, some bravery may be required if one is to break free from the siren call of stuff.

## DOORBUSTER SPECIALS

The shopping scene has certainly deteriorated since I was a teenager. In the last several years there have been several shopping melees around the world that have caused injuries and, on a couple of occasions, deaths:

> In 1996, in Frederickton, New Brunswick, three hundred people who were infected with Tickle Me Elmo fever waited outside a Wal-Mart store for five hours, then, when the doors opened, trampled a store employee so badly that he was sent to the hospital.

> In December 1998, Furbys were the hot toy of the consumer season. From coast to coast, customers lined up in the wee small hours of the morning in order to purchase one of the talking furballs. Two shoppers were injured in a stampede at a store in Nazareth, Pennsylvania; a thirteen-year-old girl in O'Fallon, Illinois, picked up a Furby and was promptly bitten on the hand by an "adult" female who wanted it; and a woman in Des Moines, Iowa, sustained minor injuries when she was trapped against a Wal-Mart door at six a.m. when the store opened and the stampede began.

The toy-induced incidents begin to seem almost quaint compared to what has occurred since the turn of the millennium:

> In November 2006, enormous crowds of video gamers, some of whom had been camping outside stores for days, waited impatiently for their chance to buy the Playstation 3 as soon as it was released. The waiting was risky: Queued-up shoppers in Kentucky were shot by someone with a BB gun, a man in line at a Wal-Mart in Connecticut was shot by robbers in the middle of the night, and there were miscellaneous minor melees all over the country.
> When the stores finally opened for business, there was a stampede at a Best Buy in Fresno, California, and a crowd in Wisconsin catapulted a nineteen-year-old into a flagpole.

> At 4:55 a.m. on Black Friday, 2008, at a Wal-Mart store on Long Island, thousands of shoppers who had been waiting since nine p.m. the previous evening for a sale scheduled to begin at five a.m., broke down the doors, crumpling the door frame and shattering the glass. The surging mob knocked down a thirty-four-year-old Wal-Mart employee and trampled him to death. Other employees who tried to aid the victim were also trampled. Eager

shoppers streamed past emergency workers who were trying to save the victim's life. At least four other people were injured. Disappointed shoppers complained bitterly when the store was closed because of the fatality.

If you are willing to trample a man to death in order to get the best possible price on a fifty-inch high-definition TV, there is a hole in your soul that is too large for even the largest television set in the world to fill.

## WHAT IS BRAVE?

I would like to believe that heroes are not immune to fear, because fear, like pain, is a signal necessary for survival. If there is no fear, can there really be courage? If there is no fear, can there be a rational, functioning mind? A small child playing on railroad tracks despite an oncoming train is not brave, he is oblivious; while an adult risking life and limb to save that child is certainly brave, because he knows enough to fear the awesome destructive power of an oncoming train.

Though it is possible to be a hero when one is afraid, it is difficult to be a hero when one's fears are irrational.

## "SICK WITH FEAR" IS ALL TOO OFTEN TRUE

Researchers are learning that fear itself is harmful to health. A study conducted by Sonia A. Cavigelli and Martha K. McClintock at the University of Chicago demonstrated that male Norway rats that were fearful and hesitant to investigate new environments died sooner than their braver littermates. The researchers tested infant rats' responses to changes in their living environments: The rats that actively explored their environment were categorized as "neophilic" (enjoying novelty), and the rats that stayed hunched up with their fur standing on end while trying to ignore their unfamiliar surroundings were categorized as "neophobic" (afraid of novelty). The researchers studied groups of littermates, pairing scaredy-rats with their brave brothers, then studied these siblings as they lived out their natural life spans. The researchers found that the fearful rats were 60 percent more likely to die at any given time than were their bolder brothers. The average life span of a fearful rat was 599 days, while the bolder rats lived an average of 701 days; none of the fearful rats lived longer than 840 days, while the longevity record for bold male rats was 1,026 days.

The researchers attributed this difference in life span to the chronic, fear-induced stress suffered by the timid rats. It is known that chronic stress can impair the immune system, cause atherosclerosis, induce diabetes, impair ovarian function, and shrink the hippocampal region of the brain. (A companion study showed that timid female lab rats died an average of six months earlier than their braver sisters. The average fearful female rat lived 493 days, while the average bold female rat lived 640 days. The female longevity records were 620 timid days versus 932 brave days.)

How does one go about becoming brave? Though researchers found that rats that were timid as infants continued to be timid throughout their lives, it would be nice to think that we humans, unlike rats, are capable of changing our mind-sets.

## HOW DO WE BECOME BRAVE?

Some may question whether bravery is really health-inducing, and suggest that being brave may actually be hazardous. But bravery and foolhardiness are not synonymous. If we discover that we are heading over a cliff, we must swerve and aim in another direction in order to save ourselves, and not just keep to our original course out of loyalty, stubbornness, or sheer momentum.

Luckily for all of us, researchers have been doing some hygienic investigating in order to determine what is truly dangerous and what is not, and they have come up with some interesting results:

1. Timidity is dangerous.
2. Dust and dirt are good for you.
3. Runny noses improve children's health.
4. Intestinal worms are your friends.

I interpret this research to mean that in this day and age, the fear of dirt is far more dangerous than dirt itself. Read on!


I was raised in a household headed by a hypochondriac, and the experience convinced me that hypochondria is one of the worst afflictions that can plague a human being. For the last forty-seven years of his life, until he died at the age of ninety-two, my poor father was convinced that he had only six weeks to live. This may sound like the punch line of a shaggy dog story, but the reality was not so funny; my father was coping with mortal terror every waking second of his life. He would not mow a lawn because "people have heart attacks while mowing lawns." He wouldn't roughhouse with his children because he was afraid the experience might kill him. He had totally unnecessary surgeries that caused very real problems.

Because one of the main themes of this book is bravery versus fear, I decided to investigate what the experts had to say about the fears that blighted my father's life. On a National Institutes of Health website, hypochondria is defined as *"a belief that real or imagined physical symptoms are signs of a serious illness, despite medical reassurance and other evidence to the contrary."* Hypochondriacs pay obsessive attention to their bodies and tend to assume that normal sensations such as the beating of the heart, or sweating, or minor health problems such as a cold, a strained muscle, or a small sore are signs of impending doom. Hypochondriacs are very, very anxious people, and unfortunately, fear and anxiety can induce many unpleasant symptoms, including increased heart rate, hyperventilation, chest pain, dizziness, excessive sweating, blurred vision, confusion, dry mouth, slowed intestinal motility (which may cause constipation and nausea), and last but not least, choking sensations. (One of my father's unnecessary operations was done because he felt as if he had "something stuck in his throat." There was nothing wrong with his throat before the surgery was done, but he certainly had something wrong for a long time afterward!) The tension induced by constant, intense fear may also cause muscle aches, trembling, shakiness, and fatigue. Just reading about it exhausts me.

I am struck by the similarity between the hypochondriac who is alarmed by the internal sensations of a perfectly normal human body, and modern society, which has learned all too well from alarmist media and advertising to be frightened by the perfectly normal manifestations of life on this planet, including the existence of bacteria, dirt, harmless invertebrates, and minor viral infections. This means we are in a constant state of near panic because we live, after all, on Earth, the dirt-and-bacteria planet.

## WHO ARE WE?

Our great-great-great-grandparents, who clearly understood that the only true reason for housekeeping is to maintain health by keeping vermin and diseases at bay, would, I think, be completely baffled by current housekeeping practices. Modern sewage systems and vaccines should be making us the healthiest, most carefree people on the planet, but we are not. We are still prosecuting our "spring cleaning" with Inquisitional vigor, as if our homes were begrimed by a winter's worth of coal dust; as if cholera, polio, typhus, diphtheria, and the Black Plague were lurking just around the corner.

It is possible that if our not-so-distant ancestors could see us, they might have trouble recognizing us as human. Researchers all over the world have been studying historical medical records, and the fruits of their research have been startling. People in the industrialized world are bigger, stronger, healthier, longer-lived, and more intelligent than their ancestors, and the differences are impressive: In 1790, the average thirty-year-old Frenchman weighed 110 pounds; his counterpart in the first decade of the twenty-first century weighs 170 pounds. During those same two centuries, the average height of Norwegian men increased by five and a half inches. The life expectancy for a baby boy born in America in 1790 was thirty-eight years; and four decades later, life expectancy in big American cities was even lower: a baby born in Boston, New York, or Philadelphia had a life expectancy of twenty-four years. By the beginning of the twenty-first century, male life expectancy had increased to seventy-three.

American men are, on average, two inches taller and 50 pounds heavier than they were a hundred years ago. During the Civil War era, the average American man was five feet seven inches tall and weighed

147 pounds, while the average American male today is five feet nine and a half inches tall and weighs 191 pounds. This means that Civil War reenactors are, for the most part, unable to use equipment that is accurate and to scale—Civil War tents and uniforms are just too small for modern-day men.

In 1861, one out of every six of the sixteen- to nineteen-year-old males who tried to sign up for the Union Army was rejected because he was disabled. This despite the fact that the army's fitness standards were quite low; a recruit with only one eye, for instance, as long as it was the right eye, was considered fit for service, and urinary incontinence was not considered a hindrance to service (perhaps the Union Army had a point; many of us wet our pants when we are terrified anyway).

Dr. Robert Fogel, of the University of Chicago, led a study of the health histories of fifty thousand Union Army veterans. These veterans had been the cream of their spindly crop of American manhood; men who, when they were inducted into the Union Army, were each in possession of two working legs, a trigger finger, and a functional right eye, and had managed to survive the war. When the researchers perused the medical records, military records, public health records, pension records, doctor's certificates, and death certificates of these outstanding specimens, they discovered that almost every single Civil War veteran suffered from a severe chronic illness for decades before finally succumbing.

What is the cause of the mind-boggling improvements in the human condition since 1800? Researchers believe that children's health in very early life is the key. Food shortages and famines were common before the Industrial Revolution; according to Dr. Fogel, one in six young adults was dangerously underweight. Prenatal and early childhood undernourishment weakened and stunted children, and made them more susceptible to diseases such as measles, rheumatic fever, typhoid, malaria, and tuberculosis. Contracting these severe diseases in early life made people more susceptible to chronic diseases such as heart disease and arthritis, which tended to strike people between ten and twenty-five years earlier than they do now.

Though stunted misery was probably the norm in Europe from the time agriculture was invented until the advent of the Industrial Revolution, physical misery was not the norm in the Americas until after Europeans arrived on the continent, carrying European diseases with them; before then, native peoples in the Americas had been quite well nourished and relatively free of epidemic diseases.

In 1524, Giovanni da Verrazano, an explorer, wrote a letter to his patron, which included this description of the inhabitants he encountered as he sailed north along the Carolina coast: "As for the physique of these men, they are well proportioned, of medium height, a little taller than we are. They have broad chests, strong arms, and the legs and other parts of the body are well composed. . . ." Later, when da Verrazano's ship reached Narragansett Bay, near what is now Newport, Rhode Island, his ship was surrounded by boats full of native people. Among those who boarded da Verrazano's ship were: ". . . two kings, who were as beautiful of stature and build as I can possibly describe. These people are the most beautiful and have the most civil customs that we have found on this voyage. They are taller than we are . . . they have all the proportions belonging to any well-built man."

The admiration was definitely not mutual. A missionary in Ontario reported that the Huron thought the French possessed "little intelligence in comparison with themselves"; furthermore, the native people agreed that Europeans in general were physically weak, atrociously ugly, and smelled terrible. The physical inferiority of the Europeans was probably caused by chronic malnutrition and disease, while the hideous stench was only what one would expect in an era when most Europeans never bathed at all.

If we compare ourselves to almost all those who came before us, we may say, with some accuracy, that we, like the inhabitants of Garrison Keillor's Lake Wobegon, live in a time and place where "all the women are strong, all the men are good-looking, and all the children are above average." We are beginning to look as if we belong here.

## ON OUR HOME PLANET

But do we *feel* as if we belong here? Over the past decade, researchers who have been investigating the "hygiene hypothesis" have found evidence that suggests that asthma, eczema, and allergies are caused by lack of exposure to dust, dirt, pets, and minor viral infections. And recent scientific studies indicate that autoimmune disorders such as ulcerative colitis, Crohn's disease, childhood-onset diabetes, and possibly rheumatoid arthritis may be caused by a dearth of intestinal parasites. This research has been widely publicized in magazines and newspapers over the years, yet there is a strong reluctance to relax our cleaning standards, perhaps partly because most of us fear incurring the disgust of our neighbors, and partly because the full force and power of industry and advertising constantly urges us on toward ever more fluorescent feats of cleanliness. Sometimes it takes a while for reality to sink in.

I am reminded of the apocryphal story about a girl who, while helping prepare a roast, asked why her mother cut both ends off the meat before roasting it. The mother replied: "It's the way it's done. My mother always did it this way." So the daughter went to her grandmother's house, and asked why she always cut both ends off the roast before cooking it. The grandmother replied, "It's the way it's done. My mother always did it that way." So the girl visited her great-grandmother, and asked the burning question. The great-grandmother replied, "I had to cut both ends off so it would fit in my roasting pan."

## LOWERED STANDARDS

While our children were small, it was a source of great wonderment to me that though my husband and I both have allergies, neither of our progeny had any allergies at all—and today both are generally as healthy as horses.

Though we invested in healthy, organic food whenever possible, and tried to stick to "natural products" for cleaning ourselves and our home, life is not perfect, and we were working with a very tight budget. But our children's limited exposure to synthetic chemicals did not explain their lack of allergies, because I was raised on an extremely healthy diet.

Our son and daughter were born in 1985 and 1988, respectively. The hygiene hypothesis first surfaced in the late 1990s, which meant that I had spent an entire decade feeling vaguely guilty about the possible effects of my relaxed housekeeping standards on my children. (But only vaguely guilty; we were having too good a time to bother with guilt.) Needless to say, the news that early exposure to dirt, dust, and dog dander may have primed my children for health made me whoop with joy. As more and more information came out, I was reminded of the scene in Woody Allen's movie *Sleeper* in which the newly awakened hero is informed that the foods that were considered health foods in the late twentieth century were actually bad for the health, and vice versa. And in several delicious instances of life imitating art, we have, in the beginning of the twenty-first century, been informed that eating chocolate should no longer be considered a vice, but rather a virtue. Dark chocolate, we are told, is full of antioxidants, lowers the blood pressure, and is good for the heart. Eggs were, for much of the twentieth century, considered bad for the heart because of their cholesterol content, but upon further examination, it was found that egg-eating generally does not affect the blood cholesterol levels of healthy people one way or the other, though it seems that eating eggs may help prevent blindness caused by macular degeneration. And the dustodons behind our doors were actually protective guardians! Of course! I'd left them there on purpose. The dog hair on the couch was carefully arranged for maximum health benefits. The overloaded, dusty bookshelves were making my children healthy and smart at the same time. My children were resilient because I'd allowed them to crawl around outside when they were babies, eating dirt, ants, and vegetables right out of the garden, exercising their muscles and their immune systems at the same time. When the toddler ate kibble out of the dog's bowl, or sucked on his sock-clad foot, he was actively acquiring beneficial microbial companions.

## WANTS VS. NEEDS

In addition to the basic mammalian necessities (clean food, water, and air), we humans, who are extraordinarily underendowed with fur, also need shelter and, in most climates, clothes. Once we get past these basic needs, we enter the realm of desire, in which differences in wealth, education, status, class, and religion create huge disparities in the way people live.

Unfortunately, deeply held beliefs can actually override the will to survive. For instance, a starving dog will happily eat anything even vaguely edible, while a starving Brahman, if offered the choicest piece of beef, would probably refuse it. I suppose I am closer to being a dog than a Brahman, for I will happily retrieve food from the floor, and have been known to salvage perfectly edible organic produce from a natural foods store's waste bin, and have subsequently fed my worm bins a little less than anticipated. I was not always such an indiscriminate feeder—I have worked hard at it, because I believe that excessive squeamishness is bad for our health and the environment.

## RELATIVE SMELLS

Many people are squeamish about smells—perhaps because advertisers and media have expended so much time and money convincing us that attractive, lovable, desirable human beings don't emit any unpleasant odors. As a result, we react with disgust and embarrassment to the perfectly natural smells that emanate from all normal human beings. Many people fight off these noisome horrors by attacking them with airborne chemical weapons that are commonly (though completely inaccurately) known as "air fresheners."

People tend to like the smells that they grew up with, no matter what those smells are. Consequently, people who grew up in the country tend to appreciate the smells of new-mown hay, freshly plowed earth, and manure, while city-bred folk tend to wax nostalgic over the smells of gasoline, exhaust fumes, and solvents. We share this love of the smells of home with many other creatures with and without backbones. Salmon follow the scents of home upstream so they can spawn in their natal waters; pigeons and migrating birds follow their noses home; so do sea turtles, newts, salamanders, frogs, and toads. Apparently, land slugs and snails also smell their way home, though each of these mollusks is the happy owner of four "noses," with one olfactory sensor located on the tip of each of its four tentacles.

Human noses are rather inadequate when compared to the olfactory organs possessed by dogs, yet research has shown that even when we are not consciously aware of smells, we still react to them. For many years it was assumed that humans did not react to pheromones (sex hormones that are detected by the olfactory organ), but researchers have recently used a bit of sly research to prove that humans do indeed secrete and react to pheromones. Dr. Geoffrey Miller, Joshua M. Tybur, and Brent D. Jordan, of the University of New Mexico in Albuquerque, published a paper in the journal *Evolution & Human Behavior* in September 2007 that delineated the effects of the menstrual cycle on strippers' tips. (That's tiPs!) The researchers asked eighteen professional lap dancers to record their menstrual periods, work shifts, and tip earnings for sixty days and a combined total of about 5,300 lap dances. Analysis of the data revealed that the dancers who were taking birth control pills (and thus not ovulating) earned steady amounts of tips throughout the study, averaging $195 per shift; while dancers who were not on the pill earned an average of $276 per shift, with much higher tips while they were fertile. Ovulating dancers earned an average of $335 in tips during a five-hour shift; $260 during the less fertile phase after ovulation; while menstruating dancers earned an average of $185 per shift.

Apparently the extra-added attractions depended upon close proximity, because the tips earned from onstage dancing remained consistent from day to day. According to the researchers, these topless (and nearly bottomless) dancers typically wear very little perfume, though they are in most other respects quite far from their natural state, being otherwise painted, curled, dyed, silicone-enhanced, trimmed, plucked, and shaven. We must assume that these ladies knew what they were doing when they chose not to wear perfume.

It seems that the way to a man's heart may be through his nose, not his stomach. And it's not just men who follow their noses. . . .

Dr. Martha McClintock has done groundbreaking work on the effects of odors on human beings. In 1971, McClintock published a study that revealed for the first time that when women live in close quarters, their menstrual cycles gradually become synchronized. McClintock concluded that this synchrony is induced by pheromones. The McClintock study was revolutionary, because when it was first published, many people still believed that humans were too lofty to have, much less be affected by, pheromones.

McClintock has headed several more recent studies in which unperfumed, undeodorized, unadulterated underarm sweat was collected from women, men, and breastfeeding mothers. Female volunteers were then exposed to these samples. Most Americans have been exposed to a virtual tidal wave of advertising meant to convince us that the smell of human sweat is disgusting, yet when the test subjects in all of these studies sniffed the unidentified "samples," they almost universally found the odors mild and pleasant. Most of the smells remained unidentified—the volunteers recognized only 9 percent of the male-derived samples and 12 percent of the female-derived samples as human odors. Of the sweat samples from breastfeeding mothers, only 52 percent were perceived as having any odor at all, and those were rated as "mild."

Some more research . . .

Claus Wedekind, of the Zoological Institute at Bern University in Switzerland, wanted to see whether humans, like laboratory rodents, prefer the smells of potential mates that are not closely related to them. Earlier studies had shown that lab mice and rats prefer mates whose immune systems are genetically very different from their own. Scientists speculated that this preference prevented inbreeding and helped produce offspring that had strong, diverse immune systems. So Wedekind recruited forty-nine female students and forty-four male students, and provided the male volunteers with clean, unscented cotton T-shirts, which he asked them to sleep in for two nights. The male volunteers were also asked to use unscented soap and shampoo, to avoid smelly foods such as garlic and onions, and to refrain from smoking and sex during those two days while they were producing experimental sweat.

The worn T-shirts were handed over to the researchers, who stuffed the shirts into plastic-lined boxes with a sniffing hole on top. Female volunteers were asked to sniff the boxes and rate the smells. Each woman rated seven boxes, three of which contained T-shirts that had been worn by men whose immune systems were similar to their own; three boxes with T-shirts that had been worn by men whose immune systems were very different from their own; and one box that contained a clean, unworn T-shirt as a control.

The women tended to prefer the scent of the men whose immune systems were the most different from their own, and many stated that the odors they preferred reminded them of their boyfriends. In contrast, pregnant mice and women who are on birth control pills (whose estrogen levels are artificially elevated) tend to prefer the smells of males whose immune systems are similar to their own. Scientists speculate that the reversal of preference occurs because it is advantageous for pregnant females to be surrounded by close relatives.

Evolutionary psychologist Steven Gangestad of the University of New Mexico took this concept a step further, and conducted a study that found that women whose immune systems were genetically very different from their male partners' seemed much happier in their relationships and were much less likely to fantasize about, or have sex with, other men, while women who were genetically similar to their partners were more likely to "wander." Men's attitudes toward sex, on the other hand, were unaffected by their genetic similarity or dissimilarity to their partners.

Charles Wysocki, an adjunct professor of animal biology at Penn's School of Veterinary Medicine, collaborated in a study in which samples of sweat were collected from the underarms of men who had refrained from using deodorant for four weeks. The sweat was blended into an "Eau de Beaucoup des Hommes," and then a little dab was applied to the upper lips of eighteen women whose ages ranged from twenty-five to forty-five. The women were told that they were testing a consumer product such as alcohol, perfume, or lemon floor wax, and were asked to rate their moods for six hours. The women reported that the odor made them happier and less tense, and none of them realized they were actually smelling sweat.

 Clean is good. But perhaps not too clean and not too deodorized.

So once one has sniffed and chosen one's mate, and the bouncing little bundle of joy has arrived, what then? In a study published in 2002, Julie Mennella, of the Monell Chemical Senses Center in Philadelphia, and a team at the University of Chicago asked twenty-six nursing mothers to wear absorbent pads in their armpits and under their bras in order to collect odors. Then, forty-five childless female volunteers were asked to smell either these odor-saturated pads, or plain control pads imbued with a random scent, four times a day. To make a long scientific story short, the smells produced by the breastfeeding mothers made the volunteer sniffers psychologically and physiologically "hot to trot."

I noticed this phenomenon in 1985, when we brought our first child home from the hospital. Two friends who came to meet the new baby went home and immediately got pregnant—one of them was unmarried and wasn't planning on having another child, and the other was married, but doctors had told her that she would not be able to get pregnant. Gentle Reader, consider yourself forewarned.

The evidence seems to suggest that the he-smells and the she-smells, when we are not told what they are, are among the most pleasant odors in the world. And the scent of home is, whether you are a man or a mouse or a salmon, also beautiful. So how have we strayed so far afield from the scents we naturally find pleasant?

## IT AIN'T THE SMELL, IT'S THE ADVERTISING

As was noticed by the original inhabitants of the Americas, long-unwashed human beings do indeed smell terrible. The porcupine is the only other creature I have encountered that smells as bad as a truly overripe human being, one who, for instance, has forgotten to bathe for several years. In fact, a porcupine's smell is startlingly similar to that of an overripe human being. But to be fair to the porcupine, I must admit that when he leaves the room, his odor leaves with him. In contrast, the smell of rancid human oils may linger long after the owner has left.

The stench of unbathed humans must have been one of the most characteristic smells in much of Europe during the time when Europeans were "discovering" the Americas. Will Durant wrote, in *The Story of Civilization*, about Europe in the fourteenth and fifteenth centuries: "Personal cleanliness was not a fetish; even the King of England bathed only once a week, and sometimes skipped. . . . In all Europe—not always excepting the aristocracy—the same article of clothing was worn for months, or years, or generations." Durant also included a quote from a sixteenth-century *"Introduction pour les jeunes dames,"* about women "who have no care to keep themselves clean except in those parts that may be seen, remaining filthy . . . under their linen." The memory of that human stench may still be haunting us, because even though we are now obsessively clean, it takes very little to make us think that we stink.

It has not escaped the attention of manufacturers, retailers, and advertisers that human beings' most powerful urges and emotions—those that drive them to seek food, shelter, and sex—are intimately connected to the sense of smell. Powerful forces exploit scents to manipulate us into buying their products, and industry researchers are working overtime to develop scents that will drive us to ever higher feats of consumerism.

## THE SCENT OF MONEY

Searching for the smells that will drive shoppers wild is the new holy grail of marketing/advertising. Many manufacturers, retailers, hotels, resorts, and spas are infusing their retail spaces and their products with specially formulated "signature" scents that are intended to attract and relax consumers, making them more likely to buy the offered products. The manufacturers are hoping that, like baby salmon in their natal stream, the smell of their "home product" will be imprinted upon consumers. The technical retail term is "branding." Someday, in order to stick to one's budget, one may need to wear nose plugs while shopping.

## THE OXYMORON PRODUCTS CONTEST

And the winner of the Oxymoron Products Contest is: "Air fresheners!" The air freshener is a shining, glorious example of a product whose use completely defies reason. Far from making indoor air "fresher," air fresheners can be dangerous when inhaled.

Air fresheners come in several different forms, among them: aerosol sprays, plug-in solids and gels, scented candles, and scented disks that, I suppose, one plays like a phonograph record. All have sneakily evocative names that are meant to make you feel as if you are being welcomed home with hugs, kisses, and homemade baked goods by family members who have been working their little fingers to the bone to make your domicile clean, comfy, and cozy; or else to make you feel as if you're on vacation. Here are the names of some of these scented products, copied right out of the U.S. government's Household Products Database: Mom's Apple Crisp; Tahitian Dream; Baking with Grandma; Evening at Home (where, exactly, would one use this product—while working late at the office?); Starlight Garden; Waterfall Scent; Crisp Breeze; Lavender Fields; Rain Garden Scent; Relax in a Hammock; Stroll Through a Garden; Wandering Barefoot on the Shore; Glistening Snow; Rainshower; and last but not least, Clean Linen.

If you are not an android, these synthetic pleasures may make you quite ill. In September 2007, the Natural Resources Defense Council tested fourteen different air fresheners. Of these, twelve contained phthalates, which some studies have linked to birth defects, reproductive problems, and hormonal abnormalities. Other ingredients included volatile organic compounds, benzene, and formaldehyde. According to the National Institutes of Health's Household Products database: "Aerosol products in general are not recommended. Inhaling vapors of hydrocarbon propellants may produce simple asphyxia with symptoms such as dizziness, disorientation, headache, excitation, central nervous system depression, and anesthesia. . . ."

One fairly typical aerosol air freshener's Material Safety Data Sheet (MSDS) shows that it contains propane, isobutane, butanem sorbitan oleate, water, and unspecified emulsifiers. Propane, butane, and isobutane are extremely flammable, may cause asphyxia, can depress the central nervous system, and can cause dizziness, disorientation, incoordination, narcosis, and nausea.

*Oooh!* What could be comfier and cozier, cleaner, fresher, and more vacationlike than a bout of central nervous system depression? And those were just the ingredients that the company was willing to disclose. They keep the identity of the sweet-smelling chemicals to themselves. Proprietary information, you know.

Why not stroll through an actual garden, holding hands with someone you love? Why not bake an actual pie? The emissions from baking even the cheapest frozen pie are certainly more benign than the exhaust from even the fanciest pie-scented candle. If you're on a diet, bake the pie, enjoy the aroma, then give the finished product to a friend or neighbor.

## PERFUME LAUNCHERS

My friend Jean refers to the industrial-strength "air freshener" dispensers that are mounted high on the walls of many public bathrooms as "perfume launchers." I suspect that these devices are mounted high up so they are harder to vandalize.

The MSDS for one model of these offensive weapons states:

> WARNING: FLAMMABLE. CONTENTS UNDER PRESSURE.
> May be mildly irritating to eyes. May be mildly irritating to skin.
> Individuals with chronic respiratory disorders such as asthma,
> chronic bronchitis, emphysema, etc. may be more susceptible to
> irritating effects.

The MSDS for this product names no actual ingredients other than benzyl alcohol; the rest are "proprietary ingredients." Benzyl alcohol is hazardous in case of skin contact and is an eye irritant. If inhaled, it can cause coughing, shortness of breath, nausea, vomiting, abdominal pain, diarrhea, headache, sleeplessness, excitement, dizziness, ataxia, coma, and convulsions.

An estimated 23.2 million Americans suffer from asthma, and the percentage of children who have asthma is rapidly increasing. As of this writing, 12 percent of children under the age of 18 have asthma. Is it really wise to conduct aggressive perfume warfare in public bathrooms?

At an event not long ago, I met two people who told me that their dogs (one dog per household) were coughing and wheezing a lot, so they took them to their respective vets. Both vets asked whether they used plug-in "air fresheners" at home. The answers were yes. The vets told them to get rid of the air fresheners. They did, and their dogs stopped coughing.

Most air fresheners contain petroleum products, and the fumes are heavier than air—thus the heaviest doses of fumes are to be found closest to the ground. Most dogs live close to the ground. So do most small children.

## LOVE PUMPKIN NUMBER ONE

Dr. Alan R. Kirsch, director of the Smell and Taste Treatment and Research Foundation in Chicago, tested the aphrodisiac effects of certain odors on humans by attaching blood flow sensors to the essential body parts, and discovered that males are more aroused by the smell of cinnamon buns than they are by perfume, and that the combined smell of doughnuts and black licorice is even more scintillating than cinnamon buns, but the most powerful love potion of all is the odor of pumpkin pie and lavender commingling. Women, on the other hand, were titillated by the smell of licorice Good & Plenty candy and cucumber.

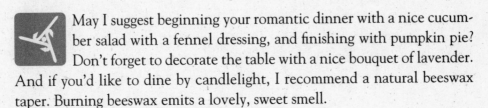

May I suggest beginning your romantic dinner with a nice cucumber salad with a fennel dressing, and finishing with pumpkin pie? Don't forget to decorate the table with a nice bouquet of lavender. And if you'd like to dine by candlelight, I recommend a natural beeswax taper. Burning beeswax emits a lovely, sweet smell.

## AD NAUSEAM

Something smells in the State of Consumerism, but it ain't the consumers, it's the advertisers, who reek of greed, duplicity, and petroleum products.

A survey showed that many people are more afraid of public speaking than they are of death! If people are afraid of looking ridiculous in front of strangers, how much more frightening is the prospect of incurring the disapproval of neighbors, friends, and relatives?

The householder must gather a bit of information and muster a bit of grit and bravery in order to decide which housekeeping practices to jettison, which to retain, and which new ones to adopt. Bravery is not always purely physical. Sometimes being brave means ignoring the disapproval of otherwise well-meaning folk and sometimes it entails speaking up in the midst of a crowd that does not agree with you.

> "Knowledge is power."
>
> —Sir Francis Bacon, 1597

## CHAPTER ONE

# The Barbarian Body

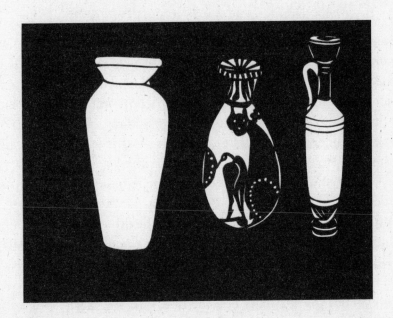

The average adult human is covered by approximately two square meters of skin that weighs between five and six kilograms (eleven to thirteen pounds). Our skin is the tough cover that protects our tender innards from hard knocks, extreme temperatures, desiccation, bacteria, viruses, fungi and yeasts, chemical and biological toxins, and ultraviolet radiation. I am happy to inhabit my skin, and delighted that I don't have to cope with frostbitten kidneys, a sunburned bladder, or dried-out eyeballs.

Undamaged skin is relatively impermeable, but in order to remain impermeable, the outer layer of the skin must be a little greasy as well as a little acidic. Dangerous, infectious microbes such as staphylococci thrive in an alkaline environment. Most soaps are alkaline, so it is fortuitous that sweat contains lactic acid, skin oils contain free fatty acids, and the beneficial microbes that inhabit the surface of our skin also produce acids.

## HEALTHY AND DIRTY

There are ten times as many microbes living in and on a human being as there are human cells that make up that body. In 2007, Dr. Martin Blaser and colleagues from the New York University School of Medicine published a study in the *Proceedings of the National Academy of Sciences* in which they identified approximately 180 different species of bacteria living on the forearms of human volunteers. Many of these bacteria are permanent residents. Said Blaser, "We think that many of the normal organisms are protecting the skin. So that's why I don't think it's a great idea to keep washing all the time because we're basically washing off one of our defense layers."

And speaking of healthily unwashed . . . health care workers in northern Minnesota occasionally find it necessary to cut the long johns off a wounded Norwegian bachelor farmer. Sometimes this is the only way to remove these undergarments because when long johns are not removed for months on end, the leg hairs become one with the fabric. But astonishingly, when the long johns are off, and all the layers of varnishlike grease and grime are washed away from the area surrounding the wound, the bachelor farmer's skin is usually perfectly smooth and healthy. Apparently even the heaviest encrustations of dirt are not, in and of themselves, conducive to disease.

Nevertheless, keeping relatively clean is still a good idea—the parasites that can settle down comfortably when the skin and hair are never washed, and clothing is never changed, may cause epidemics: Fleas can transmit bubonic plague, and lice can transmit typhus. But unlike Europeans during the Dirty Centuries, when many people wore their raiment continuously until it rotted and fell off, most people who live in modern industrial societies clean themselves often enough to avoid harboring these dangerous pests.

THE BARBARIAN BODY   29

## GOOD AND DIRTY

It can be quite difficult to remove the tenacious smell of rotting food waste that soaks into my hands when I give my vermicomposting bins a big feeding. No matter how thoroughly I scrub with soap and water, the smell of slimy garbage lingers. After trying many things, including citrus solvent, Simple Green, vinegar, and baking soda, I have discovered that the only thing that removes the lingering odor of slimy garbage is a thorough scrubbing with good, clean dirt.

I have long been a firm believer in the benefits of good, clean dirt. Over the years, this belief has amused many people who think "good clean dirt" is a paradox. But if you are outdoors with no access to washing water, and your hands are sticky, sappy, greasy, or otherwise soiled, rubbing clean dirt on your hands and then rubbing them together until you have removed as much of the dirt as possible before wiping your hands on your pants is, as far as I am concerned, preferable to remaining sticky, slimy, or stinky, and also preferable to using any type of "waterless antimicrobial hand sanitizer."

## TOWELED DRY

News broke recently that a large part of the germ eradication that is accomplished by hand washing actually occurs when the hands are briskly towel-dried; the friction removes a lot of bacteria that are still hanging on after the washing part of the operation is over. This provides scientific proof that young males who bathe perfunctorily, then wipe most of the dirt off on their mothers' towels, are getting just as healthily clean as are the more fastidious family members who wash their dirt down the drain before leaving the tub or shower. (I suggest dark brown towels for young males, or, if you live in a red clay area, rust-colored towels.)

Those horrible, deafening "electric hand dryers," because they create no friction, probably do not reduce the germ load on hands. (I've never managed to completely dry my hands using one of these machines. They are so slow and so loud that I inevitably end up wiping my hands on my pants.)

## CLAY

One ancient Egyptian version of soap was a paste containing clay or ash, which was often enhanced with perfume; another was a mixture of animal fats and vegetable oils mixed with alkaline salts. Humans have been smearing clay on their skin, or soaking their entire bodies in hot mud springs, for millennia.

Geologists, geochemists, microbiologists, and pharmacologists at Arizona State University and at the University of Buffalo in New York are investigating the antimicrobial properties of some types of clay that the French have been using on wounds for centuries. This research was inspired by a French doctor who reported that a poultice of a green, iron-rich volcanic clay from France was an effective treatment for Buruli ulcer, a devastating flesh-eating bacterial disease that is common in western and central Africa. (*Mycobacterium ulcerans*, which causes Buruli ulcer, is related to the bacteria that cause tuberculosis and leprosy.) Antibiotics are only effective very early in the course of the disease, so before the French clay treatment was discovered, surgical removal of the infected area or limb amputation was the most common treatment.

The researchers pitted clay against several types of dangerous bacteria, including *Mycobacterium ulcerans*, *Salmonella typhimurium*, streptococcus, *Escherichia coli*, *Pseudomonas stutzeri*, and *Staphylococcus aureus* (including the antibiotic-resistant MRSA strain). They found that one type of French clay, $CsAgO_2$, killed almost all of the bacteria—and what it did not kill outright, it inhibited. Even antibiotic-resistant strains of bacteria succumbed readily to the clay. Further studies showed that mixing a small amount of the clay in with sewage sludge killed all the bacteria in the sludge. Rossman Giese, professor of geology at the University of Buffalo, stated, "Nothing in the sewage sludge will grow in it."

A word of caution: The researchers tested many different types of clay, and though they found several with antibiotic properties, they found many more that did not kill bacteria. Some types of clay actually encouraged the growth of bacteria, so one should not automatically assume that just slapping any old clay on a wound is going to speed the healing process. (If you have an infection, go to the doctor!) But as microbes continue to gain the upper hand (or flagellum?) over antibiotics, the use of healing clays will probably become much more common.

Here are a couple of online retailers that sell cleansing clays:

*Mountain Rose Herbs:* www.mountainroseherbs.com
*Snowdrift Farm:* www.snowdriftfarm.com

## BEAUTIFUL LIKE THE TAJ MAHAL

Archaeologists in India have been fighting a long, desperate battle against the corrosive effects of acid rain, polluted air, and visitors' body grease on the Taj Mahal. In the early twenty-first century, researchers reading a sixteenth-century Mogul record of Indian buildings discovered that mud packs were commonly used to clean and preserve marble buildings. The archaeologists decided to try the technique, so they gently brushed layers of mud on the marble walls of the Taj Mahal, allowed it to dry, then rinsed the dried mud off. The mud pack effectively absorbed the disfiguring and corrosive black and yellow impurities from the marble, leaving it clean, white, and shining. Tests have shown that the concoction pulls sulfates, carbonates, and body grease right out of the marble. K. K. Muhammed, the head of the Agra branch of the Archaeological Survey of India, who is in charge of protecting the Taj Mahal from the corrosive effects of pollution, said: "We have analyzed the marble and feel quite happy now that it is withstanding pollution. This breakthrough has attracted attention from other archaeologists looking for ways to preserve their monuments."

If it's good enough for the Taj Mahal, it's good enough for me!

## SOAP ALTERNATIVES

### Washing Clays

There are quite a few washing clays available on the Internet. Some, like fuller's earth, which the ancient Romans used to clean wool, are white and contain very few minerals, whereas mineral-rich clays, such as the French green clays or the Moroccan green Rhassoul clay, have been used in mud packs and baths and for washing hair and skin for millennia. Clay tends to attract oil, so clay washing works quite well for oily skin and hair.

My daughter has had excellent results using Rhassoul clay packs on her face to control acne. I don't leave the clay on my dryer, more mature skin, but it does work nicely when used as a soap substitute—I just wet my skin, spoon a little dry clay on my hand, add enough water to make a wet paste, scrub my skin with the paste, then rinse.

If your skin is very dry, scrubbing with vinegar rather than soap will clean your skin without drying it out, and the vinegar will preserve the skin's natural and necessary acidity.

## WATER CONSERVATION IN THE BATH

Microfiber refers to the exceptionally small size of the fibers in a fabric, not to the composition of those fibers. Microfibers can be spun of either polyester or rayon. Fabrics that are knitted of microfiber can hold up to seven times their weight in water; they are also exceptionally good at absorbing oils. These characteristics make microfiber cloth quite useful for cleaning purposes.

I gave my new microfiber washcloth a real workout one morning, just to test it. First, I gave myself a sponge bath by scrubbing with the microfiber cloth and plain hot water (except for the stinky bits, which I washed with a regular washcloth and soap). The microfiber removed all the oil from my skin and left me squeaky clean and almost dry. Of course, one has to rinse the cloth very well in very hot water afterward in order to remove the body oils.

This bathing technique would be good for camping, as well as for people whose skin does not tolerate soap well or who are sporting medical devices that must be kept dry. Reducing the amount of water used for bathing is also not a bad idea for denizens of an overpopulated planet with rapidly diminishing freshwater resources.

## GET DIRTY, THEN GET CLEAN

They say that in order to feel pleasure, one must first experience pain, and in order to experience happiness, one must first experience sadness. I would argue that it is impossible to feel real joy in being clean if one is never dirty.

When my husband and I first started our organic landscaping business, we often had to stop at our local grocery store on the way home from work. Landscaping without machinery is an extremely sweaty, dirty activity, and the other après-work shoppers gawked as if they had never before in all their born days encountered a fellow human being who was wearing muddy work clothes. We found this quite amusing. But the pleasure we felt when we got home and simmered ourselves in our bathtub, while our newly purchased chicken roasted in the oven, was exquisite.

I strongly recommend that every able-bodied person spend at least a few days somewhere that lacks bathing facilities. Make sure that while you are there, you get good and dirty and sweaty. Once you've been really dirty, getting clean will never feel quite the same again.

### SOAP

When you are actually, rather than virtually, dirty, soap is often called for. The vast variety of natural soaps on the market give the modern consumer an almost bewildering array of choices. Because we don't like to spend hours in the store making decisions, our family has been very happily using Dr. Bronner's Liquid Soap for years. Bronner's castile soaps are vegetable oil–based and made of all-natural, organic ingredients. These soaps are so highly concentrated that we always dilute a new bottle half and half with water as soon as we bring it home.

We have discovered that the type of soap we use makes a real difference in our bodily comfort. We use peppermint soap only in the summer, when its cooling effects are most welcome; during our frigid Minnesota winters, we switch to the much warmer and blander almond soap.

## OLIVE OIL AND STRIGIL

The Romans didn't use soap at all, but rather rubbed olive oil all over their skin, then scraped the oil off—along with dirt, grease, sweat, body oils, and dead skin cells—with a metal scraper called a strigil. The Romans also used a type of clay called sapo to clean their skin.

The ancient Romans spent hours in the baths every day exercising, bathing, socializing, rubbing themselves with olive oil, and then scraping it off. The Roman baths sounded like so much fun that I was inspired to try a few things myself. My first experiment was to rub olive oil on my face and let it sit for a few minutes. My deplorable lack of a strigil led me to use a butter knife to scrape the oil off my face. My skin felt very happy afterward, so I decided that my husband and I should spend some time oiling each other and then scraping each other off.

We bought a silicone spatula, a loofah sponge, and a frosting spreader (a long, thin, metal spatula) and tested them. We gently "shaved" the oil off our faces using the frosting spreader as if it were an old-fashioned barber's straight razor. The silicone spatula was completely unsatisfactory for removing oil, so it was relegated to kitchen use. The loofah did what a loofah does. A credit card proved far too rough and unpleasant. No doubt a genuine strigil would be more effective, but we have to make do with what's available in our native era. We did not reach consensus. I loved the smooth feel of the metal spatula shaving off the oil, while Walt preferred the rougher feel of the loofah. But either way, our respective skins were very happy with the results.

If your skin tends to be dry, an olive oil treatment will make it feel and look better. Here are some suggestions:

1. Oil is very slippery. Put a nonskid mat on the floor of your tub or shower before you start. (Our mat resembles AstroTurf and is meant for scrubbing our feet.)
2. If you are actually dirty because you have been gardening, fixing the car, mucking out the stable, feeding the composting worms, or cleaning the chicken coop, you will probably want to wash yourself as usual with a washcloth and soap before you grease up.
3. If the only "dirt" you are sporting is that which you have manufac-

tured yourself, you can probably get away with washing only the "stinky bits" with soap and water. Rinse off the soap, then apply olive oil all over.

4. Scrape the oil off with the dull blade of your choice, or scrub it off with a loofah or bath scrubber. Be gentle! You are trying to remove the oil, not your outer layer of skin.

5. Rinse, then towel-dry.

## BODY BRUSHING

Several years ago I read a little account of the benefits of brush massage, also called dry-skin brushing. According to some practitioners, dry-skin brushing increases circulation, stimulates the immune system and the endocrine glands, removes toxins, rejuvenates the skin, and exfoliates dry skin cells. I thought it sounded like fun.

Though everything I have read about dry skin brushing recommends natural bristle brushes, I bought a pair of brushes that featured thick, round-tipped nylon bristles sprouting from air-cushioned bases. My husband and I tried them out on each other that evening, and have been enjoying those brushes enormously ever since.

While writing this book, I purchased a soft natural boar-bristle hairbrush for research purposes and used it for body brushing. The brush was far too stiff to be pleasant. A long-handled bath brush proved less harsh.

If your main reason for doing body brushing is to remove dead skin cells, you should probably invest in a long-handled bath brush with natural bristles. If you are aiming for sheer bodily bliss, however, I recommend a hairbrush with a cushioned pad and round-tipped nylon bristles.

The brushing technique is simple: Start at the extremities and work inward, toward the heart.

## COSMETICS

Even undamaged skin is not perfectly impermeable. Many substances can be absorbed through the skin, and depending upon the particular substances and the physiological makeup of the particular individual, each of these toxins may or may not be metabolized and neutralized, and may or may not affect the absorbee's health. But there is no doubt that the cosmetic choices we humans have made over the millennia have often had profound effects on our health.

  ELEMENTAL COSMETICS

Products concocted solely of naturally occurring substances can still be quite dangerous. It seems that nothing could be more natural than elements— the building blocks of all matter in the known universe. Yet many of these natural materials are extremely dangerous, including arsenic (As), cadmium (Cd), chlorine (Cl), chromium (Cr), lead (Pb), and mercury (Hg).

Kohl, the iconic eyeliner of the ancient Egyptians, was made by grinding green malachite, galena (lead ore), and other lead-containing minerals into a powder, then blending the powder with oil or fat. The Egyptians also used galena as a makeup base. (Kohl is still on the market, though because it is used around the eyes, it is illegal even in the United States.)

Women in ancient Greece also used white lead–based or mercury-based face paints. Galen, the great Greek physician, noted: "[W]omen who often paint themselves with mercury, though they be very young, they presently turn old and withered and have wrinkled faces like an ape."

Queen Elizabeth I used ceruse, a white, lead-based face powder, to maintain her fashionable pallor. Unfortunately, applying lead to the skin on a regular basis will inevitably result in lead poisoning. It is commonly believed that Elizabeth died of lead poisoning.

But we know better now. Or do we?

## ANCIENT HAIR DYE

The ancient Egyptians used henna (a nontoxic but permanent dye made from the leaves of the henna plant) on their hair, skin, and fingernails. Other Egyptian hair-darkening ingredients included the blood of a black ox; the ground horn of a gazelle; a donkey's liver, well rotted, then mixed with lard; or a mouse, cooked, allowed to rot, then mixed with lard.

The ancient Greeks and Romans often used a dark stain made from walnut hulls to color their graying tresses. The Romans also darkened their eyebrows with soot or charred ants' eggs. All of these natural dyes were perfectly harmless, but unfortunately, the Greeks and Romans also used lead acetate to color their hair, and the practice has continued until the present day.

## MODERN HAIR DYE

When a lead-based hair dye is applied to the hair, the interaction between lead ions and the keratin in hair yields black lead sulphide, which gradually but permanently darkens the hair. The modern version of Grecian Formula contains lead acetate and is advertised as a product that "Gradually restores lost color to graying hair . . . naturally." Part of this product's appeal is that it darkens the hair very gradually, so the change is less obvious.

Howard Mielke, a toxicologist at Xavier University in Louisiana, published a study in 1997 that showed that even when used as directed, lead-acetate hair dyes spread from a user's hands to whatever surfaces he touched. Mielke found that these hair dyes contain four to ten times more lead than is allowed in housepaint.

The only way to be sure that the hair dye you are using is lead-free is to read the label—products and product names come and go, but dangerous ingredients are forever.

## LIPS AS RED AS LEAD

In September 2007, the Campaign for Safe Cosmetics, a consumer group, bought red lipsticks in Boston; Hartford, Connecticut; Minneapolis; and San Francisco, and had them tested for lead. The independent laboratory that conducted the tests found that eleven of the thirty-three lipsticks tested contained lead levels that exceeded 0.1 part per million, which is the FDA's limit for lead in candy. It is unlikely that the cosmetic companies are purposefully adding lead to their lipsticks; the lead is probably a naturally occurring contaminant in mineral-based colorants.

L'Oréal's Color Riche "True Red" had the highest lead levels of the lipsticks tested, with 0.65 part per million. L'Oreal released a statement stating that "All the brands of the L'Oréal Group are in full compliance with FDA regulations." (According to the Campaign for Safe Cosmetics, the FDA has not set a limit for lead in lipstick.)

It is indisputable that lead is a natural substance, but it is equally indisputable that it is a very dangerous one.

The European Union has banned the use of lead in cosmetics and has listed it as a known human reproductive toxicant, a neurotoxicant, and an environmental toxin, and has warned that exposure to lead causes cumulative effects. In fact, lead is so toxic that there is nary a bodily part or system that is not damaged when exposed to it.

Canada has followed the European Union's good example and has banned the use of lead and lead compounds in cosmetics. Unfortunately, the U.S. Food and Drug Administration (FDA) has approved the use of lead as a color additive in cosmetics. Title 21—Food and Drugs, Chapter I, Part 73, Subpart C—Cosmetics Section 73.2396:

> Lead acetate: (c) Uses and restrictions. The color additive lead acetate may be safely used in cosmetics intended for coloring hair on the scalp only . . . (e) Exemption for certification. Certification of this color additive for the prescribed use is not necessary for the protection of the public health and therefore batches thereof are exempt from the certification requirements of section 721(c) of the act.

Lead acetate is simply lead that has been dissolved in acetic acid (vinegar). The pickling process makes this poisonous element easier to use as a hair dye but does not reduce its toxicity, and unfortunately, lead acetate has a sweet taste that may make it attractive to children and pets.

## MERCURY

One ancient Roman version of lash-lengthening mascara was made by beating baby mice into old wine until it formed a creamy salve. This interesting concoction would have been far less injurious to one's health than are many modern formulations.

The saying "mad as a hatter" refers to the mercury poisoning suffered by the unfortunate people who used mercury while processing beaver fur into felt to make top hats in the nineteenth century. Mercury compounds have long been used as fungicides, antiseptics, and disinfectants and until fairly recently were commonly used as preservatives in a wide variety of products. While most commercial uses of mercury have been discontinued, mercury compounds are still used as preservatives in some liquid medical products. Mercury-based preservatives include: thimerosal, phenylmercuric acetate, phenylmercuric nitrate, mercuric acetate, mercuric nitrate, merbromin, and mercuric oxide yellow.

The U.S. Food and Drug Administration prohibits mercury as an ingredient in cosmetics, except as a preservative in eye cosmetics. Skin-lightening creams that contain mercury are already illegal in the United States, but they often end up being imported anyway. These creams contain large amounts of mercury and are extremely dangerous; they can cause permanent skin damage, neurological damage, mercury poisoning, and liver and kidney damage. The only sure way to avoid permanent damage caused by imported over-the-counter skin-lightening creams is to completely avoid using these products.

In January 2008, the great state of Minnesota became the first state in the Union to prohibit the sale of all mercury-containing cosmetics, including mascara, eye liners, and skin-lightening creams.

## COSMETIC INGREDIENTS THE ANCIENT EGYPTIANS WOULDN'T RECOGNIZE

The ancients, having entirely neglected to build chemical plants, did not have access to our astounding variety of factory-produced cosmetic ingredients, so they had to make do with a finite collection of naturally derived ingredients. Things have changed since then.

According to the FDA, there are over 10,500 different ingredients that are used in cosmetic products, and more than 89 percent of those ingredients have never been evaluated for safety. The agency's regulation for cosmetic ingredients is: "a cosmetic manufacturer may use almost any raw material as a cosmetic ingredient and market the product without an approval from FDA." In contrast, the European Union's Cosmetic Directive prohibits the inclusion of any cosmetic ingredients that can cause, or are suspected of causing, cancer, mutations, or reproductive damage. The EU's strict safety standards are based on the "precautionary principle." The U.S. government's safety standards might perhaps be dubbed the caveat emptor principle. (Let the buyer beware!)

But the FDA has not completely fallen down on the job; it has limited the use of nine chemical ingredients in cosmetics. (Why ban just nine ingredients? one may, and my editor did, ask. I don't know why. Perhaps a secret FDA tribunal convened and decided that in order to placate the howling, chemophobic mob, they needed to ban some ingredients, and eventually decided to ban one ingredient for each of the nine Muses.) Here is the complete list of banned or restricted ingredients:

Bithionol
Halogenated salicylanilides
Chloroform
Methylene chloride
Hexachlorophene (HCP) (limited to 0.1%)
Mercury compounds (can only be used as a preservative in eye area cosmetics provided no other effective and safe preservative is available for use)
Chlorofluorocarbon propellants (prohibited in cosmetic aerosol products to protect the ozone layer)
Vinyl chloride– and zirconium-containing complexes (banned only in aerosol cosmetic products).

In contrast, the European Union has banned over a thousand ingredients that are suspected of inducing health problems. Perhaps countries that guarantee health care to all their citizens have a vested interest in protecting their citizens' health.

SYNTHETIC CHEMICAL INGREDIENTS

A large number of the ingredients that the FDA does not regulate are synthetic chemicals. Even though many of those substances are quite dangerous, reading a list of chemical names does not tend to pack an emotional wallop for those of us who are not chemists.

Here is a tiny list of some of the most common synthetic beauty chemicals:

## Phthalates

*Description:* Used as solvents for fragrances. Used as plasticizers in flexible polyvinyl products.

*Habitat:* Commonly found in fragrances; perfume; deodorant; nail polish; in hair care products such as shampoo, cream rinse, hair spray, hair gels and creams, and hair dyes; in skin creams and lotions; and wherever synthetic fragrances are found.

*Hazards:* May damage the liver, kidneys, and reproductive organs. May cause cancer. Suspected hormonal disrupters. (According to the Material Safety Data Sheets for many of these chemicals, their potential chronic health effects are mostly unknown.)

*Legal range:* Phthalates are very commonly found in cosmetics in the United States and in Third World countries. Some phthalates have been banned in the European Union.

## Glycol Ethers

*Description:* Solvents used as antifreeze and in paints, adhesives, dyes, inks, and cosmetics.

*Habitat:* Commonly found in nail polish, deodorant, perfume, and other scented beauty products.

*Hazards:* Causes dermatitis and at very high doses can cause liver, kidney, and reproductive damage.

*Legal range:* Very common in the United States.

## Formaldehyde

Compounds that release formaldehyde (paraformaldehyde, benzyl hemiformal, 2-bromo-2-nitropropane-1,3-diol, 5-bromo-5-nitro-1,3-dioxane, diazolidinyl urea, imidazolidinyl urea, quaternium-15, DMDM hydantoin, sodium hydroxymethyl glycinate, and methenamine).

*Description:* Preservative.

*Habitat:* Commonly found in nail polish, shampoo, eye shadow, mascara, blush, foundation, and other cosmetics.

*Hazards:* Probable human carcinogen, may cause birth defects. Causes respiratory problems, exacerbates asthma. May be toxic to the kidneys, liver, skin, and central nervous system.

*Legal range:* Common in cosmetics in the United States. Banned in the European Union.

## Hydroquinone

*Description:* Skin lightener; inhibits the production of melanin.

*Habitat:* Skin-lightening products. Hydroquinone is on the U.S. Environmental Protection Agency's list of Inert Pesticide Ingredients of Toxicological Concern.

*Hazards:* Causes irreversible skin damage, swelling, and permanent discoloration.

*Legal range:* Found in cosmetic products aimed at the African-American community. Banned in the European Union.

### CAVEAT EMPTOR

The citizens of ancient Egypt, Greece, and Rome tended to be quite interested in health, hygiene, cleanliness, and beauty, and used a wide variety of natural ingredients to beautify their skin. People who are accustomed to modern cosmetics may find many of these ingredients to be amusingly crude and even disgusting.

The Egyptians often used honey on their skin, which, though sticky, probably would not be considered disgusting by most people. The Roman poet Ovid described much more exotic skin-beautifying concoctions, including wrinkle cream made by steeping the fronds of maidenhair fern in the urine of a young boy; and skin masques that contained kingfisher, mouse, or crocodile dung; deer antlers; placenta; bone marrow; genitalia; bile; calf, cow, bull, or mule urine—all nicely blended with goose grease, honey, and/or vinegar. Pliny the Elder (Roman historian, A.D. 23–79) documented skin care practices that included treating diaper rash with a salve made of old urine blended with ash from burnt oyster shells; and restoring the color and texture of damaged skin with salves that included the lungs of sheep, the ash of an immolated green lizard, a snake's skin boiled in wine, pigeons' dung in honey, the white part of hens' dung kept in oil, bat's blood, or hedgehog's gall in water. An ancient Roman recipe for preventing ingrown hairs included a hedgehog, the fluid part of a spotted lizard's eggs, and the ash of a salamander or the slime of snails. An itch could be relieved with dog's blood or with a lotion made of the brain of a horned owl mixed in saltpeter.

It is completely obvious and goes without saying that no one living in the modern world would use or even touch cosmetics that contained such unsavory materials.

Or would we?

## THE ORGANIC ICK LIST (MODERN)

Here are a few of the nonsynthetic items from a ninety-two-page-long list compiled by the Canadian government. The list is an inventory of substances found in cosmetics that were on the market between January 1, 1987, and September 13, 2001.

Starting with the least disgusting examples and moving downward:

Avian collagen (probably chicken gelatine); ovum; gallbladder of snake; *Bombyx mori* oil (fat extracted from silkworm caterpillars); Mucoglycoproteic complex (mucus, possibly snail mucus); hydrolyzed animal thymus; hydrolyzed spleen; blood; bone marrow; heart extract; muscle extract; spinal lipid extract; embryo extract; hydrolyzed liver; lung extract; colostrum extract (colostrum is the first milk produced by a new mother); urine; tallow (animal fat); skin extract. Human placenta extract; umbilical extract; ovarian extract; testicular extract. (Note: A hydrolyzed substance is one that is combined with water.)

Unfortunately, the list also includes extracts taken from endangered animals, including *Cornu rhinoceri* (rhinoceros horn)—rhinoceroses are endangered, and trade in rhinoceros products is illegal in most countries; sea turtle oil—according to the Sea World website, all eight species of sea turtles are listed as threatened or endangered on the U.S. Endangered and

Threatened Wildlife and Plants List. It is illegal to harm, or in any way interfere with, a sea turtle or its eggs.

The ancient Egyptians would recognize many of these "modern" cosmetic ingredients, so perhaps we should stop congratulating ourselves about how far we have progressed.

The European Union's Cosmetic Directive "prohibits the use of cells, tissues or products of human origin from use in cosmetic products marketed in the EU" because they "are liable to transmit the CJD (Creutzfeldt-Jakob disease), human spongiform encephalopathy, and certain virus diseases." The E.U. and Canada also prohibit the use of bovine tissues and ingredients in cosmetics. In 2005, the FDA finally banned the use of some bovine materials, but as of 2009 still had no policy regulating the use of human tissues in cosmetics.

Scientists believe that spongiform encephalopathies are caused by exposure to prions. The FDA's somewhat cavalier attitude toward cosmetic safety is rather puzzling, because its supposed mission is to protect the public health.

Studies have shown that it is easy to infect laboratory mice with scrapie (a prion disease that originates in sheep) by lightly abrading a mouse's skin—without drawing blood—and applying scrapie prions to the roughened area. Scrapie, like all other known prion diseases, is inevitably fatal.

The U.S. Centers for Disease Control and Prevention's Biosafety Agent Summary Statement on Prions states that prions cause neurodegenerative diseases in humans and animals. There is no known treatment for prion diseases, and neither irradiation, boiling, dry heat, nor chemicals will deter or inactivate prions.

## FORESKIN CREAM

The "waste" from newborns' circumcisions is eagerly sought by laboratories that use foreskins to culture skin that can be used to help heal burn victims and diabetics who have developed skin ulcers. The foreskins are also ground up and used in extremely expensive skin creams and injectable collagens that help aging beauties maintain their assets. (One brand of cream that contains pulverized foreskins costs more than $150 per ounce. Cosmetic companies want to maintain their assets, too.)

## OVERACTIVE PRODUCTS

### Full of Bull

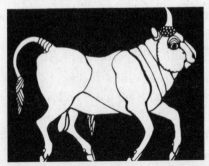

In 2007, a British manufacturer of hair care products introduced an innovative new hair treatment called Aberdeen Organic Hair Treatment, which is guaranteed to make the hair shine in a way that other hair treatments cannot. The £85.00 treatments take forty-five minutes to complete, and their main ingredient is bull semen. It seems to me that the main ingredient used in this hair treatment is easily at hand (excuse the pun) for quite a large percentage of the population. I think I would rather not have quite such an intimate (and expensive) relationship with a strange male, especially one of a different species, no matter how pretty my hair might look afterward.

Semen contains prostaglandins (very potent compounds that regulate the body's response to hormones) as well as hormones, including testosterone, estrogen, prolactin (which stimulates milk production), and luteinizing hormone (which is involved in egg cell formation in females). Though exposure to hormone-rich substances is not necessarily dangerous to adults, whose mature bodies are already producing large amounts of hormones, it is not a good idea to expose young children—whose bodies normally produce almost no sex hormones—to hormonally active materials no matter how natural or unnatural the origins of those materials. When very young children are exposed to sex hormones, the results can be truly horrifying.

### A REALLY BAD HAIR DAY

Hair care products that are "formulated for dry, fragile hair" often contain hormones or placenta. These products are targeted directly at the African-American community. African-American infants and toddlers are much more likely to develop breasts and pubic hair than are other young Americans, and several case studies have suggested that there is a connection between the use of hormonally active personal care products and these cases of frighteningly premature puberty.

A study conducted by Su-Ting Li of the Child Health Institute in Seattle, Washington, suggests that nearly half of African-American parents use these beauty products, and most of these parents also use them on their children. Perhaps not coincidentally, nearly half (48.3 percent) of African-American girls enter puberty by the age of eight, while only 14.7 percent of their white counterparts are afflicted by precocious sexual development. Chandra Tiwary, the former chief of pediatric endocrinology at Brooke Army Medical Center in Texas, said: "I believe that the frequency of sexual precocity can be reduced simply if children do not use those hair products."

Some researchers also suspect that hormonally active beauty products may contribute to young African-American women's elevated risk of breast cancer. The type of breast cancer that strikes African-American women tends to be extremely aggressive and difficult to treat, so those who develop breast cancer are much more likely to die of the disease than are white women.

Grown men are not safe from these products either. An article published in the *Journal of Endocrinology* in 1984 recounted the cases of two men, ages forty-eight and fifty-four, who used hair lotions that contained estrogens. Both men developed breasts and impotence. Fortunately, unwanted developments usually go away after men stop using the hormonally active product.

Why are these things still on the market? An embryo and its mother need a placenta, but the rest of us are much better off without. And there are good alternatives.

## CURLY HAIR CARE

The amount of curl in any specific hair depends upon the shape of the hair. Straight hair is perfectly tubular, wavy hair is a slightly flattened tube, while curly hair is more severely flattened. The kinkiest hair is nearly flat and is ridged, like curling ribbon.

Those of us who have extremely curly hair (such as my entire family) know that curly hair tends to be dry and frizzy. Shampooing makes it even drier. Try this instead.

## HORMONALLY ACTIVE HAIR CARE

Any "personal care product" that lists the following ingredients on its label may be hormonally active and thus potentially dangerous:

Placenta

Placental extract

Placental enzymes

Human placental extract

Hormone(s)

Hormone constituents

Estrogen

Estrogenic hormone constituents

## CURLY HAIR CREAM RINSE WASHING

Wet hair completely.

Massage scalp gently but firmly with your fingers.

Spray distilled white vinegar on your scalp and massage it in. This will clean your scalp and keep it from itching.

Apply nonhormonal cream rinse to your scalp and massage it thoroughly into your hair. Brush it gently through your hair to distribute it evenly, and work out the tangles.

Rinse.

Dry gently with a towel.

Do not brush or comb your hair once it is dry unless you are trying to achieve that Bride of Frankenstein, I-just-stuck-my-finger-in-the-light-socket look. (If you dry-brush your hair, apply ghoulish makeup, and then open the door very, very slowly on Halloween, you can actually scare trick-or-treaters right off your porch.)

## REALLY CURLY, REALLY DRY HAIR OLIVE OIL WASHING

If your hair is still dry and frizzy even after you have washed it with cream rinse rather than with shampoo, try washing it with olive oil.

Ingredients for Olive Oil Hair Wash

> *Olive oil*
> *Cheap vodka (If you want your hair to be lightly scented, steep a sprig of lavender, rosemary, or other pleasant-smelling herb in the vodka for a week before mixing it into the oil wash.)*
> *Water*
> *8-ounce plastic bottle*

Pour 2 ounces of olive oil and 1 ounce of vodka into an 8-ounce bottle. Add water until the bottle is full. Cap the bottle.

Follow the directions for Cream Rinse Washing, but use the Olive Oil Hair Wash instead of cream rinse. Shake the Olive Oil Hair Wash well before using. Oil and water do not stay mixed for very long.

## STEROIDS

An article published in the *American Journal of Pediatrics* in 1999 told the tale of a two-year-old boy who suddenly grew hairier, more virile, and developed acne. The boy's father, a bodybuilder, had been using a testosterone cream as part of his bodybuilding regime for two months. Apparently the boy had absorbed enough of the hormone from his father's skin to launch him into extremely premature maturity. The father stopped using the steroidal cream, and within a few months his son's precocious virility receded.

## WE'RE ALL SIMILAR UNDER THE SKIN OR CARAPACE

Botanically based pesticides and antimicrobials, which biodegrade, are preferable to synthetic chemicals, which can build up in the environment. But even though botanical pesticides are safer for the environment, they are not necessarily safe for use on humans. Many plants—for example, lavender, rosemary, thyme, tea tree, and oregano—produce fragrant oils that help protect the plants from herbivorous animals and insects. Some of these plant oils are quite biologically active and can affect insects' reproductive systems, development, or metabolic pathways. Unfortunately for human beings, we are biochemically, metabolically, and immunologically quite similar to insects (so similar, in fact, that many scientists have begun using insects as research models for many types of human disease), and these similarities may account for the discouraging effects that pesticides can produce in us.

Tea tree oil (also known as melaleuca or leptospermum) has been found to be a potent antimicrobial and antifungal, and also kills lice, ticks, and termites. Using tea tree oil in everyday products such as shampoo, toothpaste, and skin lotions is probably overkill. Perhaps tea tree oil should be saved for special occasions such as tick, lice, flea, and fungal infestations, and it should probably never be applied full strength to anyone's skin.

Lavender oil is also antimicrobial, antifungal, and insecticidal. I am quite fond of lavender, and own several potted specimens, but the concentrated essential oil, like other concentrated substances, is probably far stronger than any of us require.

Our health depends upon the health of our symbiotic bacteria. Using antimicrobials, even pretty-smelling botanical ones, on a daily basis may upset the microbial balance of our skin and create job openings for pathogenic bacteria.

## LAVENDER AND TEA TREE BREASTS

An article published in the *New England Journal of Medicine* in February 2007 related the sad story of three otherwise completely healthy, normal little boys who suddenly and inexplicably developed gynecomastia (they began to grow breasts). The boys, who were unrelated, were four years, five months old; ten years, one month old; and seven years, ten months old. All three boys were brought to Clifford Bloch, a pediatric endocrinologist, who did some sleuth work and determined that the only thing the boys had in common was that they had all been using soaps; skin lotions, balms, or creams; shampoos or hair styling products that contained lavender oil and/or tea tree oil. He told the boys' parents to stop giving these products to their sons, and once the boys stopped using these products, the gynecomastia disappeared within a year. Interestingly, the seven-year-old boy had a fraternal twin who used the same skin lotions but not the lavender-scented soap, and did not develop gynecomastia.

Afterward, researchers from the National Institute of Environmental Health Sciences (part of the National Institutes of Health) tested the effects of lavender oil and tea tree oil on human breast cancer cells and found that these oils have estrogenic and antiandrogenic properties that stimulated the growth of estrogen-sensitive breast cancer cells. A paper published in the February 2007 issue of the *New England Journal of Medicine* stated: "This report raises an issue of concern, since lavender oil and tea tree oil are sold over the counter in their 'pure' form and are present in an increasing number of commercial products, including shampoos, hair gels, soaps, and body lotions. Whether the oils elicit similar endocrine-disrupting effects in prepubertal girls, adolescent girls, or women is unknown. Since gynecomastia is labeled idiopathic (of unknown origin) in approximately 10% of men, one might speculate that unidentified exogenous sources of endocrine-disrupting chemicals may contribute to the onset or progression of the condition, or both, in such patients." In plain English, this means that they believe it is possible that using products that contain lavender oil or tea tree oil may make men grow breasts.

## NATURALLY ENHANCED—LOVE THE SKIN YOU'RE WITH

Hormonally active beauty preparations can be dangerous because the skin contains receptors for several steroid hormones, including the sex hormones estrogen, androgen, and progesterone. When these hormones and hormone precursors are absorbed, they affect the entire body.

It can be a serious problem when very young children absorb sex hormones through their skin. When consenting adults get to know each other in the biblical sense, those skin-mounted hormone receptors come in handy.

Adults, both male and female, produce testosterone, the hormone that makes people crave sex. Testosterone is best known as the hormone that makes men look and act like men. It is less well known that testosterone is produced by both males and females (though in far smaller amounts by females).

Testosterone creams are often prescribed for women who have lost their appetite for sex. Thinking about testosterone skin creams made Cameron Muir, a psychologist at Brock University, in Ontario, Canada, wonder about the role of the skin during sex. He began researching the effects of sex hormones that are released in body fluids such as saliva and sweat, and discovered that testosterone is sweated out of male armpits during sex but not during regular old exercise. According to Dr. Muir: "the amount of testosterone I found in underarm secretions is very close to the amount that doctors will prescribe to women to enhance their libido. You've heard the term hot sweaty sex . . . in an embrace, women are typically shorter than men, the nose goes somewhere near the underarm region. So if you take an evolutionary perspective on this, if you're a male and you want future reproductive opportunities, it pays to dose a female with testosterone through a bit of sweat from your underarms. . . . We'd like to look at saliva as well because we kiss—a big long drawn-out wet kiss—and there's a lot of steroid hormones in saliva."

## THE APPLE OF LOVE

"Sweat is the perfume of lovers
sweat is the best perfume . . ."
    —Geggy Tah, lyrics from "Special Something"

The path to true love is not necessarily sanitized and deodorized. Ascending the heights of sensuality sometimes causes one to get sweaty.

For several months I searched for confirmation that the fabled "Apple of Love" really existed. I had read vague reports that young maidens in Shakespeare's day used to hold pieces of peeled apple in their armpits, then present them to their paramours as a fragrant remembrance. Eventually, Nick, my intrepid research assistant, found an article in the 1899 *Journal of American Folklore* that included the following: "To make a girl love you, take a piece of candy or anything she is likely to eat, and put it under either armpit, so that it will get your scent."

And then, at last, a confirmed sighting of the Apple of Love! In an article titled "The Sexual Significance of the Axillae," published in the journal *Psychiatry* in 1975, author Benjamin Brody wrote: "In contrast, it has been the custom in rural Austria (and may persist in that slow-moving culture) for the girls to keep slices of apples in their armpits during dances, perhaps as a natural deodorant. At the end of the dance the girl would present the slice to her favorite partner and he would gallantly eat it."

Of course I had to try it. So on a bitterly cold morning in early December, I sliced up a Honeycrisp apple, and peeled and cored two smallish slices that were just thick enough for structural integrity. I dutifully kept those apple slices clamped into my armpits and reread Mark Twain's "Diary of Adam and Eve" while on the stair stepper, in order to speed up the process of imbuing the apple slices with sweat. There is a lot about apples and romance in that story.

It was rather difficult to function with apple slices in my armpits, and at about two o'clock I lost my grip on the larboard apple slice while I was battening down the hatches in the chicken coop in anticipation of a night that was forecast for twenty below. The apple slice ran aground at about the level of my lowest rib because my shirt was tucked in. When I got back in the house, I pulled the piece of apple out of my shirt. The slice was amazingly smooth, dry, and nonsticky, and really still smelled just like an apple.

I spent half the day smelling like an apple before I began to smell like myself again. (Those lively Austrian girls may have been on to something.

Apples really are effective armpit deodorizers.) After about seven hours of holding my arms close to my sides, I removed the apple slices, zipped them into a freezer bag, and put the bag in the refrigerator. When my husband got home, he gallantly ate some of the Apple of Love. So did I, because I wouldn't want to make him do anything I wouldn't do. The apple was still crisp but was completely saturated with my sweat, and the taste hit me hard in the back of the palate, as if I were eating a slice of very strong Brie cheese. This part of the palate, perhaps not coincidentally, coincides with the location of the vomeronasal organ (which senses pheromones) in many mammals.

 Incubating an Apple of Love for just half an hour induces a much milder, less explosive experience.

There are reports, from different parts of the world, of men wearing handkerchiefs in their armpits while they dance, then waving the male-scented fabric under the noses of women they are interested in. Scented hankies are obviously less troublesome than creating an Apple of Love, but who wants to eat a hankie?

Many people find the fragrance of expensive perfume much more pleasant than the smell of human sweat. This is quite understandable. Perfume is a sexy smell, too. It should be. Many expensive perfumes and colognes contain either civet, musk, or castorium. Civet is an oily substance produced in the glandular pouch that is located between the genitals and anuses of civet cats, which are native to southern Asia and Africa. Musk is an oily substance produced in a small bag or sac that is attached to the prepuce (foreskin) of the male musk deer of Central Asia. Castorium is produced in the perianal glands of beavers (*Castor sp.*). These expensive animal-derived oily substances "fix" the fragrance of perfumes, slow their evaporation, and make the perfume last much longer.

If the thought of musk, civet, or castorium is too much for you, perhaps you should stick to perfumes that are formulated with ambergris, a rare and expensive fatty, waxy substance that is vomited forth by sperm whales that roam the Indian Ocean and the southern Pacific Ocean.

Civet, musk, and ambergris are far too expensive to use in cheap perfume, dish liquids, laundry detergent, dryer sheets, shampoo, or children's bubble bath. Cheap synthetic fragrances contain phthalates, some of which, as was mentioned earlier, are suspected hormone disrupters.

## A WITCH'S BREW

After sailing hither and yon on the fast currents of the Internet, chasing down information about the modern State of Beauty, I have arrived at the following conclusion: The modern business of beauty is far dirtier and more disgusting than anything the ancients could ever have imagined. The witches in *Macbeth* might have cackled with delighted recognition at the list of macabre ingredients found in modern cosmetics. They might also have been quite enchanted by the amount of hormonal havoc wreaked by modern "beauty products" on the environment as well as on innocent children.

One of the liver's many functions is to break down toxins and render them harmless. When toxic substances are absorbed through the skin, they bypass the liver and may remain dangerous far longer than they would if ingested. If you want to be healthily beautiful inside and out, avoid applying substances to your skin that you would not be willing to eat.

Now that we've got the skin covered, what about the rest of the Barbarian Body?

Here are a few useful websites with information about cosmetic safety:

The Environmental Working Group: www.ewg.org/reports/skindeep

European Food Safety Authority: www.efsa.eu

The EU Directive: www.safecosmetics.org

Campaign for Safe Cosmetics: www.safecosmetics.org

## CHEWING GUM WILL MAKE YOU SMART

The ancient Greeks chewed gum from the bark of the mastic tree, which grew in Greece and Turkey. Chewing mastic helped clean the Greeks' teeth and sweetened their breath. The Mayans chewed chicle, the sap of the sapodilla tree. American Indians in New England chewed spruce gum. Archaeologists have found five-thousand-year-old lumps of black tar with the impression of human teeth in them in bogs in Germany and Scandinavia, and ancient Britons chewed birch bark gum.

In modern times, chewing gum has often been looked down upon as "low class." The gum-snapping, fast-talking, wisecracking, lower-class gal has been a fixture in many a movie and stage play. Now twenty-first-century researchers are beginning to prove that gum chewers are not just faster talkers, they are faster thinkers as well.

Andrew Scholey, of the University of Northumbria in Newcastle, U.K., pitted gum-chewers against non-gum-chewers, and the gum-chewers won. During high-stakes, twenty-minute tests of short- and long-term memory, the gum-chewers prevailed by margins of 24 percent in the immediate word recall test and 36 percent in the tests of delayed word recall. Gum chewers also displayed superior spatial working memories.

In 2000, Japanese researchers using magnetic imaging witnessed a huge surge in activity in the hippocampus, an area of the brain that is important for memory, when their research subjects chewed. Chewing also increases heart rate and makes more oxygen and nutrients available to the brain.

## CAVITIES ARE CONTAGIOUS

Saliva helps clean the teeth and buffers the acids that can cause tooth damage. It also contains proteins and fats that help protect tooth surfaces, and calcium and phosphorus, which can help remineralize the teeth.

Chewing gum helps increase salivation and thus speeds up the tooth-cleaning and rebuilding process. Researchers have found that sugarless gum that contains xylitol is especially beneficial because xylitol reduces the population of cavity-inducing *Streptococcus mutans* bacteria, and also helps prevent the transmission of S. *mutans* from mouth to mouth. Mothers commonly infect their children with the S. *mutans* bacteria. (Studies have shown that mothers who chewed xylitol gum during the first two years of their children's lives were less likely to infect their children with the S. *mutans* bacteria, and their children had a greatly reduced incidence of cavities in later life. The xylitol gum was much more effective at reducing S. *mutans* than was treatment with either fluoride or with chlorhexidine, a chemical antimicrobial that is often added to mouthwashes.)

Xylitol also reduces the accumulation of plaque on the teeth. Other studies have shown that chewing xylitol gum reduces the incidence of cavities in schoolchildren, even in those who eat large amounts of regular candy.

- Xylitol is a sugar substitute that is made from birch and other hardwood trees. It is also found in small amounts in fruits and vegetables.
- Xylitol is one of the many foods that are safe for humans but not for dogs: Xylitol causes a rapid and potentially fatal drop in dogs' blood sugar levels and can also severely damage the canine liver. Keep all xylitol-containing items out of the reach of canines; eight pieces of sugarless gum may be enough to kill a sixty-five-pound dog, and a couple of pieces could kill a small dog.

(Note: Xylitol ingested in large amounts tends to have a laxative effect. Consider yourself forewarned. Everything in moderation.)

Recent research has found that chronic oral infections may lead to heart disease, lung disease, and stroke, and pregnant women who have oral infections may be more likely to go into premature labor and produce low-birth-weight babies. The insurance companies obviously haven't been paying attention to the research, nor to the surgeon general's 2000 *Report on Oral Health*. Surely it would be cheaper to pay for routine dental care rather than for increasing numbers of premature infants, heart attacks, strokes, lung disease, and diabetes. Two routine dental checkups per year may set you back as much as $600, but according to the Healthcare Cost and Utilization Project, the average bill for a heart attack in 2004 was $16,200, and the average bill for a stroke was $11,100. But not all heart attacks are alike: A 2007 article in the *Oakland Tribune* detailed the financial woes of a Vallejo woman whose heart attack had cost a whopping $701,995.

Kiss someone who has good teeth today!

## CLEARING THE EARS

Colds and allergies can block the eustachian tubes, which drain fluid from behind our eardrums. Excess fluid leads to a buildup of pressure and causes pain. Chewing gum can help relieve the pressure and pain of an ear infection. Note: Do not give gum to very young children, who may choke on or swallow it.

## ALL LIT UP BUT STILL CLOGGED

Ear candling is an "ear clearing" technique used in holistic or folk medicine. The thin, hollow cones made of beeswax-impregnated cloth are widely available in "alternative" stores. Proponents claim this is an ancient technique that has been practiced for millennia in many different parts of the world. Some manufacturers of these devices refer to them as "Hopi" ear candles, and continue to do so even though the Hopi tribe has repeatedly asked them to stop, since ear candling is not and never has been a Hopi practice.

In order to use the ear candle, the earwax-afflicted patient lies on his side. The candle is then inserted into the ear and lit. The candle is allowed to burn down until it threatens to set the patient's hair on fire, at which point it is extinguished. The suction caused by the flame is supposed to draw earwax up and out of the ear.

Health Canada conducted laboratory tests that showed that ear candling "produces no significant heating or suction in the ear canal." However, there is plenty of evidence that ear candling produces significant risk of injury. A survey of 122 ear specialists, published in 1996 in the medical journal *Laryngoscope*, found that these doctors had treated thirteen cases of burns, seven cases in which wax from an ear candle had dripped into the ear and blocked the ear canal, and one case of a punctured eardrum caused by an ear candle.

Ear candles burned in ears produce earwax-colored residues that are chemically identical to residues produced by ear candles that have been stuck in a glass container and allowed to burn down. This residue is not earwax. Apparently the only thing that an ear candle really removes is money from the consumers' pockets.

Perhaps it is just as well that ear candles do not actually suck all the wax out of ears, because ear specialists advise that earwax is there to waterproof your ear canal and protect it from infection. If you remove the earwax, you are changing the acidity of your ear canal and are asking for an infection. Leave it alone. (You don't wipe the moisture off your eyeballs, do you?) If you really think you have impacted earwax, visit your friendly neighborhood ear specialist.

## KEFIR

Kefir is a dairy product that is produced by fermenting milk with kefir grains, which are translucent, resilient communities of fungi and bacteria that peacefully live together in a symbiotic clump. It is believed that kefir was first produced many centuries ago by shepherds in the Caucasus mountains of Russia; it has been touted as a health food ever since.

A couple of years ago my friend Connie gave me some kefir grains so I could grow my own. I loved my delicious new "pet" and immediately began reading up on it. I learned that kefir is ridiculously salubrious. The friendly bacteria found in kefir grains and kefir include sixteen varieties of lactobacilli, two types of lactococci, *Streptococcus thermophilus*, *Enterococcus durans*, two leuconostocs, and three acetobacters. Over a dozen species of yeasts or fungi have also been found in kefir. This intense biological activity qualifies kefir as a valuable and very complex probiotic food.

Research has shown that kefir inhibits the growth of pathogenic bacteria, stimulates the immune system, inhibits the growth of cancerous tumors, and has antiviral and antifungal properties. In 2005, Brazilian researchers K. L. Rodrigues, L. R. G. Caputo, J. C. T. Evangelista, and J. M. Schneedorf published a paper in the *International Journal of Antimicrobial Agents* that showed that kefir killed several species of staphylococcus in open wounds in the skin of laboratory rats. The rats whose wounds were treated with kefir healed more quickly than did the rats who had been treated with an antibiotic salve. In 2007, Korean researchers M. Y. Lee, K. S. Ahn, O. K. Kwon, M. J. Kim, M. K. Kim, I. Y. Lee, S. R. Oh, and H. K. Lee published a paper showing that feeding kefir to asthmatic mice reduced asthma attacks. The researchers stated that the kefir exhibited strong anti-inflammatory and antiallergenic effects.

As soon as I read the words "kefir has antifungal properties" I decided to begin an experiment. I have suffered from a nasty toenail fungus on my left foot for more than two dozen years. The infection appeared just after Walt and I got married (weddings are horribly stressful!). I tried various treatments, but antifungal pills made me sick, soaking my foot in vinegar did nothing except make my foot cold, and antifungal ointments weren't effective. I even tried smearing my toenails with Vick's VapoRub (recommended by *Consumer Reports*) for over a year. The VapoRub seemed to be working for a while, but then the fungus returned, so I discontinued the treatment.

I soaked my foot in kefir every day for a month; then the holidays descended upon us, and all semblance of order vanished from my life. I only managed to soak my foot about once a week, and our offspring were both disgusted and charmed (in order of birth) when I allowed the dogs to clean my foot and lick the bowl after soaking my toes. I figure that our canines' innards were more than capable of dealing with my used kefir. Their foraging habits are far from genteel.

Despite my lackadaisically intermittent kefir treatments, my toenails seem to be growing out fungus-free. I will continue my weekly kefir soaks and won't rush to judgment. I've been through this before, and as they say, it ain't over till it's over. Since both canine saliva and kefir have been reported to have antifungal properties, if my toenails grow out fungus-free, there may be some question as to which liquid did the trick, the saliva or the kefir. But I'm sure there are many itchy-footed people out there who will be able to apply both dog slobber and kefir to their feet.

Note: Just drinking kefir is apparently enough to cure some people (my sister, for instance) of foot fungus.

## SPIT ON IT

Modern researchers have learned that human saliva has antibacterial and antifungal properties. We can probably safely assume that canine saliva shares these properties, which may account for the several reports of miraculous cures of athlete's foot and toenail fungus that have apparently been effected by dogs licking their owners' fungus-infested feet.

Our three-year-old friend Ailee has chronic skin problems that she inherited from both parents. Her cute little cheeks are frequently red and raw from eczema. I gave her parents some kefir grains and asked them to try applying kefir to Ailee's skin the next time she got a rash. Ailee obligingly broke out in a rash soon thereafter. According to her dad, Jim, her little arm was covered from shoulder to wrist by a rough rash that felt like sandpaper. Ailee was anointed with kefir cream several times a day, and the rash was gone within a week. This was the first time in her short life that one of these rashes had healed in less than a month. Jim said that all the other lotions and ointments they tried on Ailee made her complain that her skin was burning. The only time Ailee complained about the kefir was when it was applied cold, right out of the refrigerator. Now Jim keeps a small jar of kefir on the counter in the bathroom.

Ailee's baby sister, Carlee, recently volunteered to help test the effects of kefir on diaper rash. The results were quite encouraging and compared favorably to the organic diaper rash ointment that Carlee had been using.

## MORAL OF THE STORY?

The Greek myth of the fierce Libyan giant Antaeus was quite popular with classical poets and artists. Antaeus, the son of Poseidon (the sea) and Gaia (Mother Earth), challenged all strangers to wrestle. Antaeus inevitably won these matches because he was invincible as long as he remained in contact with the earth, his mother. Antaeus won so many matches that he was able to build a temple to Poseidon out of the skulls of his erstwhile opponents. The giant was finally defeated by the hero Herakles: "Hercules held fast in his arms the sweating earth-born Libyan, when he found the trick and snatched him upon high, and left him no hope of falling, nor suffered him to touch even with his foot's extremity his mother earth" (Statius, *Thebaid*, Roman epic first century A.D.). And this, from Ovid's *Metamorphosis*: "I [Herakles] uprooted fierce Antaeus from his mother's nourishment."

Unfortunately, looking and smelling unnaturally good can cost us more than money. We are all children of the Earth, and when we remove ourselves too completely from our source and her teeming multitudes of microbes, we suffer.

CHAPTER TWO

# At the Barbarian's Table

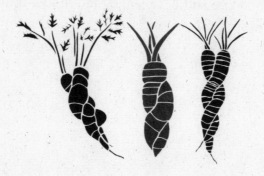

"An army marches on its stomach."

—Napoleon Bonaparte

And food must traverse the stomach in the right direction and at the right speed, or the mission will fail.

Not only are we what we eat, but as we eat, we are remaking the planet in our own image. As our collective diet becomes less balanced and less local, our farmlands are also losing their balance and resilience, and in some instances are simply disappearing under an avalanche of development. If the people who are growing our food for us on the other side of the planet ever decide that they would rather eat that food themselves, we will be in big trouble. Unfortunately, it has always been much easier to make a parking lot by paving over a fertile field than it is to make a fertile field by breaking up a parking lot.

## SUBSIDIZED CROPS

The U.S. government has been subsidizing American agriculture ever since the Great Depression, when it became obvious that keeping American farmers in business and on their land was crucial to the welfare of the country. Funny how we seem to have forgotten that.

Keeping farmers on the land is, of course, vitally important. A country that cannot feed itself is terribly vulnerable to disruption. Unfortunately, crop subsidies were not originally designed to bolster *all* food production, and even now a relatively small variety of crops are subsidized. The most heavily subsidized crops are corn, wheat, and soybeans.

A U.S. Department of Agriculture (USDA) crop subsidy publication states that since 1996, "policy initiatives are focused on increasing demand through trade liberalization, expanding new uses, enhancing crop yields and quality. . . ." (Translation: The USDA is concentrating on increasing the demand for the same old commodity crops.) The same publication states that "Under the North American Free Trade Agreement (NAFTA), Mexico immediately reduced its soybean tariff on NAFTA partners to 10 percent, and phased it out completely by 2003. With reforms in Mexico's domestic crop support programs, imports have virtually displaced domestic soybean production, with nearly all imports coming from the United States. As a consequence, U.S. soybean exports to Mexico have doubled since 1993 to over $900 million." Apparently we don't mind driving Mexican farmers off their land. But we do seem to mind when displaced Mexican farmers migrate north, looking for jobs. Neither, according to the USDA, do we seem bothered by the fact that "The largest 9.7 percent of farms in terms of gross receipts received 59.5 percent of all government payments in 2005," nor do we seem troubled by the fact that since the passage of the 2002 Farm Act, direct fixed payments "are based on historic acreage and yields and are considered 'decoupled,' that is, not based on current production or prices. Direct payments are projected at $5.25 billion over the remainder of the 2002 Act." Nor is our government concerned about the fact that "Producers are free to plant most crops on base acreage, with some limitations on planting fruit and vegetables. Producers can even elect to leave the land idle. Thus, these payments are considered to be minimally production- and trade-distorting." These payments may not be especially "production- and trade-distorting," but they do distort many other things.

There have been some rather bizarre consequences to these "decoupled" payments. According to a July 2006 article in the *Washington Post*, Mary Anna Hudson, who lives in the formerly rural River Oaks neighborhood in Houston, has received direct crop subsidy payments totaling $191,000 over the past decade. Houston surgeon Jimmy Frank Howell, as of the 2006 suburban nonplanting season, had received $490,709 in crop subsidies. And suburbanite Donald Matthews, who lives in a brand-new luxury home in the heart of rice country in El Campo, Texas, receives about $1,300 in annual "direct payments" because years ago rice was grown on his eighteen acres. Mr. Matthews is an asphalt contractor and does not grow crops. "I don't agree with the government's policy," said Matthews, who wanted to give the money back but was told it would be given to other landowners. "They give all of this money to landowners who don't even farm while real farmers can't afford to get started, it's wrong."

An article published in the *San Francisco Chronicle* in December 2001 told the tale of billionaire Charles Schwab, of the stock brokerage firm, who at that time owned 1,500 acres of duck- and goose-hunting land in the middle of rice fields. Mr. Schwab's share of crop-subsidy loot amounted to $564,000 in the year 2000. In 2005, the federal government handed out more than $25 billion in farm aid, which was almost 50 percent more than was paid to families on welfare.

## EAT YOUR VEGGIES

Despite the urgings of doctors, mothers, and the U.S. Department of Agriculture, most Americans are still not eating their vegetables. In 2007, researchers in Baltimore analyzed data from government surveys conducted from 1988 to 1994 and from 1999 to 2002, and found that approximately 62 percent of Americans ate no fresh fruit and 25 percent ate no vegetables at all. Vegetable consumption actually decreased during the period of the surveys.

A 2005 report released by the Centers for Disease Control and Prevention (CDC) showed that Americans who earned more than $50,000 per year ate more fruits and vegetables than did people who earned less; college graduates ate more fruits and vegetables than did those with less education; and people who were not overweight ate the most fruits and vegetables, while the most obese people ate the least.

The U.S. government recommends that adults eat two cups of fruit and three cups of vegetables each day. One might assume that a government that wants its citizens to eat more produce would try to help make produce more affordable. However, upon perusing the 2008 version of the farm bill, a thoughtful observer would probably conclude that the U.S. government is not ready to put its money where its mouth is.

Like all its predecessors, the new farm bill declares that fruits, vegetables, and tree nuts are "specialty crops" that "are not eligible for direct support under USDA's farm commodity price and income support programs." The farm bill restricts participants from planting fruits and vegetables on acreage that is already part of the commodity program. In other words, the asphalt farmer we met earlier in this chapter would lose his $1,300 annual commodity payment if he planted fruit or vegetable crops rather than a lawn on his eighteen-acre estate.

In 2007, a Minnesota farmer named Jack Hedin ran afoul of the commodity system when he expanded his acreage by renting twenty-five acres from two neighboring farmers. Mr. Hedin grows watermelons, tomatoes, and vegetables to supply local natural foods stores and local customers. In an op-ed article published in *The New York Times* on March 1, 2008, Mr. Hedin wrote that everything was going well until early July, when, as they say, the tomatoes hit the fan:

> That's when the two landowners discovered that there was a problem with the local office of the Farm Service Administration, the Agriculture Department branch that runs the commodity farm program, and it was going to be expensive to fix.
>
> The commodity farm program effectively forbids farmers who usually grow corn or the other four federally subsidized commodity crops (soybeans, rice, wheat and cotton) from trying fruit and vegetables. Because my watermelons and tomatoes had been planted on "corn base" acres, the Farm Service said, my

landlords were out of compliance with the commodity program.

Typically, a farmer who grows the forbidden fruits and vegetables on corn acreage not only has to give up his subsidy for the year on that acreage, he is also penalized the market value of the illicit crop, and runs the risk that those acres will be permanently ineligible for any subsidies in the future. (The penalties apply only to fruits and vegetables—if the farmer decides to grow another commodity crop, or even nothing at all, there's no problem.)

Mr. Hedin suddenly owed his landlords an additional $8,771 in order to make up for their lost subsidy payments for the year. Hedin explained the reason for this seemingly irrational farm policy in this way: "Why? Because national fruit and vegetable growers based in California, Florida and Texas fear competition from regional producers like myself. Through their control of Congressional delegations from those states, they have been able to virtually monopolize the country's fresh produce markets."

Commodity price supports keep the prices of commodities such as corn, soy, wheat, and rice low; fresh, perishable foods are quite expensive in comparison. Perhaps it is not coincidental that poor people are more likely than the rich to suffer from a lack of fresh fruits and vegetables.

## SCHOOL LUNCHES

The National School Lunch Program was instituted in 1946 in order to ensure that schoolchildren got at least one nutritious meal each day. Children who could afford to pay, did, while children who could not afford to pay were given free lunches.

Section 2 of the School Lunch Act defines its purpose: "It is hereby declared to be the policy of Congress, as a measure of national security, to safeguard the health and well-being of the Nation's children and to encourage the domestic consumption of nutritious agricultural commodities and other food. . . ."

The goal of encouraging domestic consumption of agricultural commodities has certainly been met. Most schoolchildren, like most other Americans, are not suffering from a shortage of commodities such as soy protein, hydrogenated soybean oil, corn syrup, or macaroni and cheese, and many of us have the waistlines to prove it.

An outstanding example of governmental hostility to vegetables occurred during the Reagan administration. In 1981, the administration had already cut the funding for the school lunch program by $1 billion (40 percent of the program's total budget) and wanted to make further cuts. The administration decided to cut another $180 million from the program by reducing the size and quality of the children's meals.

The Reagan administration's recommended cost-cutting proposals included officially classifying ketchup and pickle relish as vegetables, thus making the condiments eligible to serve as the vegetable component of a school lunch. Soon thereafter, a group of Democratic senators invited reporters and photographers to watch them as they ate school lunches, each of which consisted of a meat-and-soybean patty, a slice of bread, a few french fries, ketchup, and a partially filled glass of milk. (Perhaps more nutritionally savvy diners might have forgone the ketchup so that they could have been allowed a lettuce leaf or a slice of tomato on their burgers.)

Soon afterward, an article published in the *Washington Post* reported that President Reagan and his budget director, David Stockman, had agreed that the guidelines should be reconsidered "due to adverse public reaction," though Stockman also stated that "The president and I both feel that the intent was sound and in step with the administration's goal to reduce regulation and return flexibility to the local units of government."

Later, James Johnson, an aide to Agriculture secretary John R. Block, defended the regulations by telling the press: "There was a great misunderstanding in the land as to how these regulations are viewed. I think it would be a mistake to say that ketchup per se was classified as a vegetable. . . . Ketchup in combination with other things was classified as a vegetable."

When a reporter asked "What other things?" Johnson replied: "French fries or hamburgers."

I'm so glad he cleared that up.

## SOY

The USDA has been quite diligent about "expanding new uses" for subsidized crops. Soybean oil now accounts for 79 percent of the edible oils used annually in the United States. Dr. Joseph Hibbein, at the National Institutes of Health (NIH), estimates that soybeans, mostly in the form of oil, now contribute up to 10 percent of the total caloric intake in the United States.

The Food and Drug Administration has gotten into the commodity promotion act as well, and now allows food companies to proclaim on their product labels that a daily diet containing twenty-five grams of soy protein may reduce the risk of heart disease.

## SOY BY ANY OTHER NAME . . .

This governmental cheerleading hardly seems necessary. Soy, in one form or another, is already an ingredient in nearly all of our processed foods, including baked goods, chips, cereals, pancake mixes, frozen foods, cookies, candy, breakfast cereals, frozen pizzas, frozen dinner entrées, packaged sauces and gravies, dips and spreads, noodle dishes, fried fast foods, chicken nuggets, fish sticks, and dairy desserts. Textured soy protein, which is made from defatted soy flour, is used to make imitation meat products such as soy sausages, burgers, franks, and cold cuts, as well as soy yogurts and cheeses.

Soy's aliases include lecithin, soy flour, vegetable oil, protein concentrate, textured vegetable protein, hydrolyzed vegetable protein, soy protein isolate, and plant sterols.

## SOY MILK

Sales of soy milk increased by 110 percent between 2001 and 2004. Silk, the most popular brand of soy milk, was America's best-selling "white beverage" in 2004, with sales that topped $400 million. Soy is very, very big business. In contrast, cow's milk, which is quite perishable, is a much more local product.

Soy milk can be made from processed soybeans, soy flour, or soy protein solids, so some soy milks are more "natural" than others, depending on how heavily processed the starting ingredient is. But no matter how natural they are, all commercial soy milks need to be sweetened in order to give them more flavor than the container they come in.

The most common method for processing soybeans uses the solvent hexane, which is a petroleum product, to extract the oil from the beans, after which the defatted protein can be processed into products such as soy flour, soy protein solids, animal feed, or soy milk.

The popularity of soy milk is soaring because 74 percent of Americans believe soy products are healthy. But is soy really wholesome?

Soybeans (*Glycine max*) belong to the legume family, which includes more than 16,400 species, many of which are not particularly friendly. The more dangerous members of this family have some very effective ways to protect themselves from predation: Some contain potent toxins that kill hungry herbivores quickly; others deploy toxins that gradually cripple the hapless animals that graze on them; some produce toxins that induce memorable pain and nausea; and yet others contain compounds that reduce fertility.

## THE HUMBLE ORIGINS OF SOY

The soybean is native to China, where it has been cultivated for more than three thousand years.

In the early twentieth century, Professor F. H. King, who had retired from service with the U.S. Department of Agriculture, traveled widely in China in order to research the techniques that the Chinese used to maintain their soil fertility. He returned and wrote the book *Farmers of Forty Centuries: Organic Farming in China, Korea, and Japan*. In the introduction King wrote: "Almost every foot of land is made to contribute material for food, fuel or fabric. Everything which can be made edible serves as food for man or domestic animals. Whatever cannot be eaten or worn is used for fuel. The wastes of the body, of fuel and of fabric worn beyond other uses are taken back to the field; before doing so they are housed against waste from weather, compounded with intelligence and forethought and patiently labored with through one, three or even six months, to bring them into the most efficient form to serve as manure for the soil or as feed for the crop." Professor King found that the vast majority of soybeans were grown as green manure to be tilled into the soil. When a crop of soybeans was actually harvested, rather than just being dug into the soil, the beans were usually ground up and then formed into large cakes that were pressed so the oil could be extracted. The defatted, pressed soybean cakes were traditionally used as fertilizer, though by the time Professor King toured China, some of the cakes were being shipped to Europe for use as stock feed and fertilizer. The only other use for soybeans that King described in detail in his book was the use of soy flour paste by cloth dyers, who applied the paste through patterned stencils, then allowed the paste to dry before dipping the cloth into vats of indigo blue. The cloth beneath the soy paste remained white while the rest of the cloth turned deep blue.

Bean curd (tofu) merited a single, passing mention. It appears that these people who wasted nothing, who ate everything that could be "made edible," ate very little of a crop they had been cultivating for three millennia. Soybeans had been cultivated for over a thousand years before someone figured out that if soybeans were cooked, processed, then allowed to ferment, they were rendered edible. These fermented soy foods, which included soy sauce, salty black beans, miso, and fermented tofu, were most commonly used as condiments to season vegetables, rice, meat, and fish.

## FEMININISOY

Phytoestrogens—estrogen-mimicking chemicals produced by plants—are found in very high concentrations in soybeans. For many years, soybean advocates have been recommending soy to menopausal women as a "natural" estrogen replacement that would help them avoid hot flashes and some of the other unpleasant side effects of menopause. Research has shown that drinking two glasses of soy milk every day for a month will shift the timing of a woman's menstrual cycle.

In 2000, the new advisory from the American Heart Association Nutrition Committee recommended that Americans eat at least twenty-five grams of soy protein daily, because soy protein lowers cholesterol levels and seems to strengthen the heart. Eating soy has also been found to reduce the incidence of breast, colon, and prostate cancer. The soy-marketing gurus are loudly trumpeting all these health benefits because soybeans are very, very big business: Biotech corporate giants such as Monsanto, Archer Daniels Midland, Cargill, Bunge, and Louis Dreyfus control the multi-billion-dollar global soybean industry. Unfortunately, dissenting voices have been speaking very softly indeed.

## HORMONAL THERAPY

Soybeans contain several different flavonoids (aromatic compounds) that can induce various distressing conditions in animals. Studies dating back as far as 1959 have shown that animals fed diets that contain large amounts of uncooked soybeans develop goiters (swollen thyroid glands at the front of the neck). In animals that haven't been fed soy, goiters are usually a sign of a thyroid disorder or an iodine deficiency. (Iodine deficiency used to be quite common in regions where iodine was lacking in the soil and drinking water, which is why most table salt in the United States is now iodized. Goiters in humans can grow to be quite large and unsightly.) The thyroid gland secretes hormones that regulate the metabolism of food and help maintain a healthy balance of calcium and phosphorus in the body. A healthy thyroid gland is necessary for the normal growth and development of juveniles. Be kind to your thyroid gland!

## SOY AND AUTISM

The incidence of autism, a developmental disorder that impairs the ability to interact with other people, has been steadily increasing in recent years. Postmortem and brain imaging studies of autistic brains have shown that their structure is abnormal, and that autism affects many major structures of the brain, including the limbic system, cerebellum, corpus callosum, basal ganglia, and brain stem. The autistic brains have irregular patterns and abnormally oriented cells that make them appear disorganized.

Some researchers suspect that there may be a link between eating soy and autism. A study conducted by Gustavo C. Román of the University of Texas, and published in the *Journal of Neurological Sciences* in November 2007, investigated the role of flavonoids (phytoestrogens) in causing autism. Dr. Román stated, "Experimental animal models have shown that transient intrauterine deficits of thyroid hormones (as brief as 3 days) result in permanent alterations of cerebral cortical architecture reminiscent of those observed in brains of patients with autism. I postulate that early maternal hypothyroxinemia resulting in low T3 in the fetal brain during the period of neuronal cell migration (weeks 8–12 of pregnancy) may produce morphological brain changes leading to autism." (Translation: Pregnant animals whose thyroid hormone levels are suppressed may produce offspring with brain anomalies that resemble those seen in autistic humans.)

Dr. Román continued: "Insufficient dietary iodine intake and a number of environmental antithyroid and goitrogenic agents can affect maternal thyroid function during pregnancy. The most common causes could include . . . maternal ingestion of dietary flavonoids or . . . antithyroid environmental contaminants. Some plant isoflavonoids have profound effects on thyroid hormones and on the hypothalamus–pituitary axis. Genistein and daidzein from soy (*Glycine max*) inhibit thyroperoxidase that catalyzes iodination and thyroid hormone biosynthesis." (Translation: Eating a lot of soy may depress the thyroid function of a pregnant animal.)

Researchers I. Carina Gillberg, Christopher Gillberg, and Svenny Kopp, of the Child Neuropsychiatry Centre in Göteborg, Sweden, studied a group of five autistic children (three boys and two girls), three of whom were born with congenital hypothyroidism, and two of whom had mothers who had been hypothyroid during their pregnancies. These researchers concluded that hypothyroidism during early fetal development might induce nervous system damage that would cause autism. (Translation: Mothers who have low levels of thyroid hormones during pregnancy may be more likely to produce autistic offspring.)

Soy-eating is rising and so is the incidence of autism. Coincidence?

## PRETTY SOYS

Trent Lund of the Department of Biomedical Sciences at Colorado State University discovered that eating soy products is a great way to prevent baldness, prostate cancer, and acne. Apparently, equol, a molecule produced in the intestine when the soy phytoestrogen daidzein is digested, binds to dihydrotestosterone (DHT), the male hormone responsible for male-pattern balding, acne, excess body hair, and prostate growth.

Men who are not enjoying their male hormones—which are responsible for men's increased body hair, decreased scalp hair, larger muscles, deep voices, thick (and sometimes bumpy) skin, heavy bones, increased metabolism, and active interest in sex—might consider eating more soy.

## VERY SLOW SWIMMERS

Dr. Lorraine Anderson, a reproductive health specialist at Belfast's Royal Maternity Hospital, was studying infertility and trying to discover why some sperm were so slow that they were incapable of reaching, much less

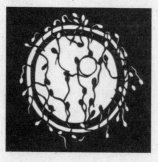

fertilizing, an egg. Said Anderson, "It doesn't matter how many sperm a man's got; if they can't get from A to B then there's little chance of reproduction." The breakthrough came when an analysis of the slow sperm samples revealed that the seminal fluid that surrounded the sluggish sperm contained phytoestrogens. The most common dietary source of phytoestrogens is soy.

Dr. Anderson also stated that if a boy eats a lot of soy while growing up, the phytoestrogens can affect the development of his reproductive tract and may lead to undescended testicles as well as to testicular cancer in later life.

## SOY IN A BOTTLE

Twenty-five percent of American infants are fed soy formula. American babies are ten times more likely to be fed soy formula than are British infants, and Israel has restricted soy formula to prescription-only status.

The U.S. government convened a panel in 2006 to evaluate the safety of soy-based infant formula. After due deliberation, the panel stated that it had "negligible" concern that the ingestion of soy formula could harm newborns and infants, even though animal studies have shown that soy can stunt growth, cause reproductive system abnormalities, and decrease fertility. The panel's official conclusion was that very few studies have looked at the long-term effects of soy formula.

Robert M. Blum, Jamie Swanson, and Jill E. Schneider of the Department of Biological Sciences at Lehigh University in Bethlehem, Pennsylvania, wondered whether soy formula could be partly responsible for the decrease in the average age of female puberty that has been observed over the last thirty years. Though the marketplace has no conscience, most scientists do, so rather than conducting their experiments on human infants, these researchers tested their hypothesis on baby hamsters. The researchers found that feeding one of the soy phytoestrogens to baby hamsters made the babies reach sexual maturity earlier than normal. Some later studies conducted on rodents and nonhuman primates yielded similar results.

## 25 PERCENT OF AMERICAN INFANTS PARTICIPATE IN A REALLY BIG EXPERIMENT

C. H. Irvine, N. Shand, M. G. Fitzpatrick, and S. L. Alexander of Lincoln University in Canterbury, New Zealand, published a study in the *American Journal of Clinical Nutrition* in 1998 in which they measured the amount of phytoestrogens ingested by formula-fed infants. The researchers recruited twenty-nine infants, four of whom were fed a soy-based formula, while the other twenty-five dined on a dairy-based formula.

Only the soy-based formulas contained detectable levels of phytoestrogens. The researchers then analyzed urine collected from the subjects' disposable diapers and discovered that only soy-formula babies excreted phytoestrogens. Soy-fed babies, no matter their age or weight, were getting a daily dose of phytoestrogens of approximately three milligrams per kilogram of body weight per day.

Very-low-dose birth control pills contain twenty micrograms of estrogen; these lower-dose pills are believed to be safer for women who are nearing menopause. Regular birth control pills contain thirty to fifty micrograms of estrogen. (A microgram equals one millionth of a gram.) If a fifty-kilogram (110-pound) woman takes the strongest birth control pills, she will be ingesting fifty-millionths of a gram of estrogen per fifty kilograms of body weight, which works out to one millionth of a gram of estrogen per kilogram of body weight. The lowest dose of phytoestrogens delivered in soy formula was three milligrams per kilogram of baby weight per day. (A milligram is a thousandth of a gram.) So the soy-formula infant gets a dose of phytoestrogens that is *three thousand times as large* as the dose of estrogen ingested by a one-hundred-ten-pound woman on birth control pills.

Are phytoestrogens really that similar to estrogen? Researchers Beck, Unterrieder, Krenn, Kubelka, and Jungbauer of the University of Natural Resources and Applied Life Sciences in Vienna, Austria, extracted phytoestrogens from red clover (*Trifolium pratense*) and soybeans (*Glycine max*) in order to evaluate their use in hormone replacement therapy. The researchers applied these extracts to estrogen, progesterone, and androgen receptors, and stated that the estrogenic activity was "in the same range as recommended for synthetic estrogens."

No one knows whether these soy-fed infants will have health problems as they mature and age. It's an experiment!

## SOY BOYS

There have, however, been studies of the prenatal effects of soy. Researchers at the Johns Hopkins Medical Institutes conducted a study in 2003, in which they fed genistein, a soy phytoestrogen, to pregnant rats. After waiting for their subjects to mature, the researchers discovered that prenatal exposure to genistein produced adult male rats with lower testosterone levels, smaller testes, and larger prostate glands than normal. The soy rats had normal sperm counts, but abnormally low sex drives.

Male human fetuses produce large amounts of testosterone between the seventh and eighth weeks of gestation. This testosterone surge masculinizes the fetus. (Female fetuses do not undergo a similar surge of hormones; they automatically develop into females because the basic mammalian pattern is female.) The customized male version has male genitalia, a male reproductive tract, and a masculinized brain that expresses male-specific behavior patterns. Laboratory studies on rodents have shown that if the male hormone is blocked during this critical time of gender development, the male pups are likely to develop genital defects such as hypospadias (abnormal positioning of the opening of the urethra) or undescended testicles.

In the late 1990s, a team of researchers in Bristol, U.K., investigated the connection between maternal diet and hypospadias. The researchers conducted detailed studies of the medical, lifestyle, and dietary histories of mothers-to-be participating in the Avon Longitudinal Study of Pregnancy and Childhood. Mothers who participated in the study produced 7,928 baby boys, 51 of whom had hypospadias. The researchers looked at every imaginable variable and found that maternal smoking, alcohol consumption, previous use of birth control pills, number of previous pregnancies, number of miscarriages, and age of mother at puberty had zero effect on the incidence of hypospadias. However, vegetarian mothers were 4.99 times more likely to produce a son with hypospadias than were omnivorous mothers. The researchers concluded: "As vegetarians have a greater exposure to phytoestrogens than do omnivores, these results support the possibility that phytoestrogens have a deleterious effect on the developing male reproductive system."

## SOY BRAINS

In 1999, the agribusiness giants Archer Daniels Midland and DuPont sponsored a conference in Washington, D.C., to explore the role of soybeans and soy products in the prevention and treatment of disease. They got more than they bargained for.

The conference was supposed to focus on the use of soy as a "natural" cure for heart disease, prostate cancer, breast cancer, osteoporosis, menopausal "hot flashes," and other chronic conditions. But the mood of the conference may have changed a bit when Dr. Lon White presented the results of the Honolulu Heart Program. The program was set up to study the health of 8,006 Japanese-American World War II veterans who were born between 1900 and 1919.

The researchers compared the dietary habits and health of these men between 1965 and 1993. According to Dr. White, the scientists found "a significant link between tofu consumption during midlife and loss of mental ability and even loss of brain weight."

The subjects were questioned about twenty-seven foods and beverages, and the data showed that those who ate more tofu tended to have impaired mental abilities. Tofu was the only consistent link between the men, Dr. White said. Brain function declined more rapidly among the tofu eaters, whose cognitive test scores "were about equivalent to what they would have been if they were five years older," said Dr. White. "Guys who ate none, their test scores were as though they were five years younger."

Three hundred test subjects died during the study, and their brains were autopsied. When Dr. White examined the brains of the tofu eaters, he saw that "the simple weight of the brain was lower."

Dr. White talked about the increasing popularity of soy foods, due to their reputation as health enhancers. The phytoestrogens, also known as isoflavones, the most talked-about compounds in soybeans, "are molecules that the soy plant makes while it's germinating to help it fend off mold and other things that attack the plant in the ground. They're plant molecules that look like estrogens but they're not natural estrogens. When they get into cells, they actually affect the metabolism of cells."

"The bottom line," Dr. White emphasized, "is these are not nutrients.

They are drugs. They will have some benefits and some negative things."

Among the attendees at the conference was Finnish scientist Herman Adlercreutz, who had been studying the effects of soy on breast and colon cancer rates. His studies in the 1980s led to an explosion of interest in soy. Adlercreutz believed that eating more soy would improve the health of Westerners. But Adlercreutz said at the conference: "I am myself frightened a little bit by all of this. There is so much we don't know."

## HIGH-FRUCTOSE CORN SYRUP

The USDA has also been wildly successful at promoting corn, another of the big commodity crops. According to Todd Dawson, a biologist at the University of California, Berkeley, corn typically accounts for 69 percent of the carbohydrates in the average American's diet, and most of those carbohydrates are ingested in the form of high-fructose corn syrup. "We're like corn chips walking because we really have a very, very large fraction of corn in our diets, and we actually can't help it because it's an additive in so many of the foods we find on the market shelves," Dawson says.

High-fructose corn syrup is both sweeter and cheaper than sugar, which is why it has become an essential ingredient in almost all sweetened processed foods, including soft drinks and baked goods, and in condiments such as ketchup and barbecue sauce.

Unfortunately, it seems that the slippery slope leading to obesity may be lubricated with soda pop. . . .

Dr. Matthias Tschöp, a researcher at the Obesity Research Center at the University of Cincinnati, led a study of the effects of sweetened water on young male laboratory mice. Four different groups of mice were fed standard laboratory mouse chow. Group A's water was sweetened with 15 percent fructose, in order to simulate an average American soft drink. Group B was given the European version of a popular soft drink that contained 10 percent sucrose. Group C was given a popular diet soft drink. Group D was given plain water. The researchers carefully measured the total amounts of food and beverage that each mouse ingested. In addition, the rodents were weighed and sent through MRI machines three times a week in order to determine their body fat and muscle percentages.

After seventy-three days of this regimen, the mice were sacrificed and analyzed. The mice who drank fructose-sweetened water had gained significantly more weight than did the mice who drank other beverages. The MRI scans revealed that this increase in weight was due to an increase in fat mass. The fructose mice piled on fat despite the fact that all the mice in all the groups had a similar caloric intake throughout the study; apparently, the mice in the fructose group had compensated for the calories in their water by cutting back on the amount of food they ate. The researchers also found that the mice who had been drinking diet soda had significantly higher blood insulin levels compared to the mice in all the other groups.

Moral of the story: If you want your pet mice to remain slim and healthy, don't give them soft drinks.

A study published by Dr. Ramachandran Vasan in the July 2007 issue of *Circulation* showed that people who drank more than one soft drink a day were 50 to 60 percent more likely to develop metabolic syndrome than were those who abstained from soft drinks. Metabolic syndrome increases the risk of developing high blood pressure, diabetes, and heart disease; some telltale signs of this syndrome include obesity, high blood pressure, an increased risk of blood clots, and insulin resistance. Dr. Vasan said: "We were struck by the fact that it didn't matter whether it was a diet or regular soda that participants consumed, the association with increased risk was present."

Type II diabetes is characterized by insulin resistance—a loss of sensitivity to insulin that leads to elevated levels of insulin in the bloodstream. In 2007, nutritional scientists at the University of Alberta were the first to discover that high insulin levels lead to a buildup of cholesterol inside blood vessels. Dr. Donna Vine and her research team studied insulin-resistant rats and found that fats linger longer in the bloodstream after a fatty meal if insulin levels are too high. Under normal circumstances, large lipid (fat) particles called chylomicrons transport fats from the bloodstream to the liver for processing. An excess of insulin hinders the chylomicrons' progress and makes them more likely to stick to the sides of the blood vessels, where they can form plaques and cause atherosclerosis and heart disease.

# IT'S NOT NICE TO MESS WITH MOTHER NATURE— DAVID VS. GOLIATH

Monsanto began its corporate life in 1901 as a chemical company called the Monsanto Chemical Works. Its first product was saccharin; other early Monsanto products included vanillin, caffeine, sedatives, laxatives, and aspirin. During a more mature phase in its corporate life the company began producing plastics, resins, fuel additives, industrial fluids, vinyl siding, antifreeze, fertilizers, herbicides (including the infamous Agent Orange, which was used as a defoliant during the Vietnam War), pesticides, AstroTurf, and polychlorinated biphenyls (PCBs). Some of Monsanto's products, including Agent Orange, were contaminated with dioxins, which are extremely toxic chlorinated compounds that are common by-products of industrial processes that use chlorine. Dioxins are persistent contaminants that do not break down in the environment; exposure to dioxins may cause many varieties of cancer and birth defects, and may damage the reproductive, endocrine, and immune systems. Fifty-six of Monsanto's former chemical plants are contaminated with dioxins and/or PCBs and have been designated as Superfund sites by the Environmental Protection Agency (EPA). Monsanto, through a series of corporate maneuvers and mergers, transferred all but one of these Superfund sites to a spin-off chemical company called Solutia in 1997. According to an article published in *Chemical & Engineering News*, Solutia filed for bankruptcy in December 2003 in order to get out from under $100 million in liabilities, including the retirement pensions for former Monsanto employees and the legal and remediation costs of dealing with contamination at Monsanto's former manufacturing plants.

Monsanto first began transforming itself from a chemical company to a biotechnology company in the 1970s. In 1981, it created a research division devoted solely to plant genetics, and it has never looked back. According to Monsanto's website: "Monsanto is an agricultural company. We apply innovation and technology to help farmers around the world be successful, produce healthier foods, better animal feeds and more fiber, while also reducing agriculture's impact on our environment."

It is a grave error to assume that a behemoth company cares about you personally, about humanity in general, or about the fate or health of our planetary ecosystem.

In 1998, Percy Schmeiser, a farmer from Bruno, Saskatchewan, was sued by Monsanto for infringing the patent on its genetically engineered Roundup Ready Canola. Monsanto claimed that Mr. Schmeiser had planted their canola seeds without paying the $37-per-hectare licensing fee. Monsanto agents had "discovered" that 320 hectares of Mr. Schmeiser's fields were growing canola plants that contained Monsanto's patented Roundup-resistant genes.

Roundup Ready crops are engineered to survive being doused with high concentrations of Monsanto's herbicide Roundup. The only reason to plant Monsanto's expensive, poison-coordinated Roundup Ready seeds is if you plan to spray large amounts of Monsanto's matching herbicide on your fields in order to decimate all green living things that are not canola.

Mr. Schmeiser had been growing canola on his fourteen-hundred-acre farm for forty years, and as farmers have been doing since farming began, had been diligently developing canola varieties that were well adapted to his particular growing conditions. In 1997, Mr. Schmeiser first discovered genetically modified canola in a ditch by one of his fields. He sprayed herbicide on the wandering canola and was surprised to find that it was unaffected by the poison. Schmeiser then did a field test by spraying Roundup on three acres of his canola crop, and discovered that 60 percent of the plants near the ditch were resistant to the herbicide. The farther they were from the ditch, the lower the percentage of herbicide-resistant plants.

In court, Mr. Schmeiser claimed that he had planted his 1997 crop with seed he'd saved from the previous year, and insisted that he had never purchased Monsanto seed. Monsanto claimed that Schmeiser had illegally bought Roundup Ready seed from local growers in 1997, then saved seed to plant his 1998 crop.

Mr. Schmeiser was particularly stubborn and tenacious. Unlike dozens of other farmers who had been sued by Monsanto for the same offense, he refused to settle out of court. Monsanto sought a total of $400,000 for damages that included patent infringement, civil damages, legal expenses, lost profits, technology fees, and punitive damages. Mr. Schmeiser's defense showed that he didn't purposefully acquire Roundup Ready seeds, didn't try to save their patented seeds for future planting, and didn't spray his canola crop with Roundup. In 2001, after a three-week trial, the Federal Court of Canada issued its judgment. Justice Andrew McKay upheld the validity of Monsanto's patented Roundup Resistant gene. The judge agreed that a farmer generally owns the genes of the seeds or plants grown on his land, except in the case of genetically modified seeds. Justice McKay ruled that no matter how the genetically engineered plants got into a field, whether the farmer planted them on purpose or the seeds fell off a passing truck, or pollen from genetically modified plants blew in from another field, Monsanto still owned the modified genes of the plants.

The Federal Court of Appeal rejected Mr. Schmeiser's appeal in 2002. Mr. Schmeiser kept trying, and his appeal was finally heard in Canada's Supreme Court, which determined that Monsanto's patent was valid, but Schmeiser could not be forced to pay anything to Monsanto because he did not profit from the presence of the Roundup Ready canola in his fields.

In 2008, Schmeiser settled his lawsuit against Monsanto out of court. Monsanto agreed to pay all the cleanup costs of removing the Roundup Ready canola from Mr. Schmeiser's fields. The agreement included the provision that Monsanto could be sued if their product contaminates his fields in the future.

In a 2007 report, the Center for Food Safety, in Washington, D.C., documented 112 patent-infringement lawsuits launched by Monsanto against farmers in twenty-seven states. According to Bill Freese, the center's science-policy analyst: "The number of cases filed is only the tip of the iceberg." Freese has been told of many instances in which Monsanto investigators have confronted farmers at their homes or in their fields, claiming that the farmers are violating a technology agreement and demanding to see their records. This is how Freese described one such scenario: The investigators will show the farmer a surveillance photo of himself and then will say, "Monsanto knows that you are saving Roundup Ready seeds, and if you don't sign these information-release forms, Monsanto is going to come after you and take your farm or take you for all you're worth." It takes a lot of guts and a lot of money to stand up to that kind of intimidation. According to the lawyers of many farmers who have been sued by Monsanto, most of their clients give up, settle out of court, and pay Monsanto for damages.

Monsanto even has a toll-free snitch number so that neighbors can inform on each other. The company has sued cooperatives as well as the owners of country stores, so don't assume that Monsanto doesn't want to hear from you even if you live in the suburbs or the city. If you suspect that your unfriendly neighbor is growing a row of corn in his vegetable garden that might contain some of Monsanto's patented genes (which is possible, since these genes seem quite mobile) you can call Monsanto's Seed Piracy number toll-free at 1-800-768-6387.

Or, if the totalitarian stench is too much for you, try calling all your local food retailers and tell them that you don't want to eat genetically modified food; then contact all your legislators and urge them to sponsor legislation to change U.S. patent laws so that they can no longer be used as implements of extortion.

## GODZILLA VS. BAMBI

Unfortunately, many impoverished farmers in Third World countries do not have the wherewithal to fight back. In India, for instance, salesmen travel from village to village singing the praises of Bt cotton, Monsanto's genetically modified cottonseed. Bt cotton is protected from bollworms because it contains genes from the insecticidal bacteria *Bacillus thuringiensis* (Bt), and these fancy seeds are also engineered to be Roundup Ready, just in case. Of course, such fine seed is expensive—costing at least twice as much as regular cottonseed—but the salesmen assure the farmers that their customers have had wonderful yields because of these superior seeds. Traditionally, Indian farmers saved their own low-tech cottonseed from year to year. Many farmers were convinced that Monsanto's seeds were truly superior, and borrowed money from banks or local moneylenders to buy the patented seeds.

If the weather was propitious and the cotton yielded well, all was well. But farming is a risky business, and it seems that Bt cotton was not as well adapted to Indian weather as are traditional cotton varieties. If his Bt cotton crop failed, the farmer ended the season with no money to pay his debt and no way to buy seed for the next crop. Many people, including Britain's Prince Charles and Dr. Vandana Shiva of India, have claimed that genetically modified crops are responsible for the alarming epidemic of farmer suicides in India. The *New York Times* reported that in 2003 alone, more than seventeen thousand Indian farmers committed suicide.

## LOWERED YIELDS AND ENVIRONMENTAL DESTRUCTION, TOO!

The environmental effect of Roundup Ready crops is quite obviously negative, because they tolerate and increase the use of the herbicide. The wholesale spraying of poisons is generally not a good thing for environmental or human health. Nearly five years of British experiments showed that crops of genetically engineered, herbicide-tolerant canola, corn, and beets caused more environmental damage than did crops of their conventional counterparts. Fewer butterflies and bees were found flying amid the genetically modified (GM) crops, and the scientists feared that there would also be a decline in the songbird population, because songbirds feed mainly upon the seeds of broadleaf weeds. These studies were the first to evaluate the environmental impact of a new farming practice before it was introduced.

If any GM crops were actually increasing crop yields and thus decreasing world hunger, perhaps we could swallow our objections and learn to live with their very considerable flaws. But so far there is no conclusive evidence that genetic engineering helps farmers increase their yields. In 2005, a rigorous independent study conducted by Ma and Subedi in the United States showed that Bt corn does not outproduce conventional corn. The researchers found that though Bt corn sometimes yielded as well as conventional corn, it never outperformed conventional corn. The yield from low-tech corn seeds was sometimes as much as 12 percent higher than the yield from the Bt corn.

After hearing from farmers that GM soybeans did not produce bumper crops, agronomist Dr. Barney Gordon decided to investigate. He conducted three years of field tests at Kansas State University, planting both GM soy and conventional soy in the same field, and found that the GM soybeans produced only seventy bushels of grain per acre, while an almost identical variety of conventional soybeans produced seventy-seven bushels per acre. Studies conducted at the University of Nebraska showed that another variety of Monsanto GM soybean yielded 6 percent less than its closest conventional relative. After the results of the Nebraska study were published, Monsanto released a statement stating that it was surprised by the size of the reduction in crop yield, but not by the fact that the yields had dropped. Monsanto said that the soybean had not been engineered to increase yields, and the issue was being worked on. I wonder whether the farmers who had spent extra money to buy GM seeds from Monsanto paid Monsanto a licensing fee for the privilege of growing the patented seed and then spent more money buying Monsanto's Roundup herbicide were surprised to learn that the seeds had not been engineered to increase soybean yields.

## GM OH, MY!

Many thoughtful people are worried about the impact of GM foods on human health, and many thoughtful people are not; there is no convincing evidence one way or the other . . . yet.

However, a study of genetically modified field peas conducted by Australia's national science agency, the Commonwealth Scientific and Industrial Research Organization (CSIRO), was abandoned in 2005, after ten years' worth of research, when tests showed that the GM peas were making laboratory mice desperately ill.

Dried, shelled field peas are used to make split pea soup, and the entire dried pea plant, peas and all, is commonly fed to farm animals. Field peas are extremely susceptible to the pea weevil (*Bruchus pisorum*), which lays its eggs on pea pods. After hatching, each larva eats its way into a pea seed, where it remains until it grows up and eats its way out of house and home. The gaping exit holes reduce the yield and value of the field pea crop, and Australian farmers must monitor their crops very closely in order to apply pesticides in time to prevent weevil infestation.

CSIRO scientists identified a bean gene that produces a protein that makes weevils starve to death, then spliced the weevilcide gene into field peas. The resultant field peas were 99.5 percent resistant to pea weevils. After some troubling results with chickens and pigs, the CSIRO scientists solicited help from researchers at the John Curtin School of Medical Research in Canberra (JCSMR). The JCSMR researchers fed groups of laboratory mice either beans, non-GM field peas, or genetically modified field peas twice a week for four weeks. Neither the bean-fed mice nor the traditional-pea mice showed any evidence of immune reactions, but the mice that were fed the GM field peas began displaying immune system reactions after two weeks of their untraditional diet, and the allergic reactions increased over time. The lungs of the GM-fed mice became inflamed, and blood tests revealed that their tiny bodies were primed to react to other food allergens. It is one thing to modify food crops so they poison invertebrates; it is quite another to modify food crops so they poison mammals. CSIRO ended the field pea program.

In 2007, 142 million acres in the United States were planted with genetically modified crops, and worldwide the figure was 282 million acres. When you eat nonorganic products that contain ingredients made from corn, soybeans, canola oil, or cottonseed oil, you are almost certainly eating genetically modified food. We are in the midst of an experiment on a rather large percentage of the population that consumes food with ingredients made from genetically modified soy, corn, and cottonseeds. Stay tuned for the results.

## SWALLOWING SMALL SEED COMPANIES

The Bayer, Syngenta, Monsanto, DuPont, BASF, and Dow Corporations are the world's largest pesticide manufacturers; among them they control approximately 80 percent of the agrochemical market. These giants have also bought out many seed companies, and these acquisitions have made DuPont, Monsanto, and Syngenta the world's largest seed companies. These companies maximize their profits by genetically engineering seeds that will only thrive when doused with chemicals produced by the home company. And their strategy is working. According to a report prepared for the United

Nations Conference on Trade and Development, global sales of agrochemicals, which include herbicides, insecticides, fungicides, and other agrochemicals, suddenly began rising in 2003 after a twenty-year-long period of stagnating or decreasing sales. Global sales of agrochemicals were estimated at US$32.665 billion for 2004, with the Big Six earning a combined share of approximately 77 percent of the market.

On its website, Syngenta describes itself as "a world-leading agri-business committed to sustainable agriculture through innovative research & technology." But the year after it was formed, Syngenta collaborated with Myriad Genetics, a biotech company in Utah, and won the race to sequence the rice genome, beating the International Rice Genome Sequencing Project—a publicly funded project that involved scientists in Japan, China, South Korea, Europe, and the United States.

Syngenta and Myriad claimed that they had mapped the approximately fifty thousand genes that make up the rice genome to 99.5 percent accuracy. Syngenta said it was willing to share its information with academic researchers, but would not put all their genome data in the public domain as a publicly financed genome project would.

Dr. Steve Briggs of the Torrey Mesa Research Institute in San Diego, California, where much of Syngenta's work was done, said, "the biggest surprise is that the overall gene architecture and sequence is nearly identical to that of cereals. This means we truly have a plant genetic blueprint."

In 2005, Syngenta submitted patents to the European Patent Office, the U.S. Patent and Trademark Office, and the World Intellectual Property Rights Organization (WIPO), seeking global patents for fifteen groups of gene sequences for rice. The patent documents ran to 529 pages, and in them, Syngenta claimed to have invented 30,000 of rice's genes. Syngenta's patent claims are also aimed at other plants, including corn, sorghum, rye, bananas, soybeans, wheat, and many fruits, vegetables, and other plants, because the company claims that most of the gene sequences that it has "invented" are identical to those in other plants and thus their patent must also extend to those plants. Syngenta's voluminous documents include an attempt to patent the "method of modulating carbohydrate, protein, fatty acid composition" (in other words, photosynthesis); the "Plant DNA involved in control of flowering time in rice . . ."; "DNA mediating phosphate uptake; protein;

transgenic plant, cereal; maize, soybean, sorghum, wheat, rice . . ."; "DNA from plant, polypeptide; plant; dicot; monocot, including cereal, rice, sorghum . . . expression of genes; progeny . . . seeds . . ."; "18 DNAs from maize, rice . . . wheat, hordeum (barley) . . . monocot, dicot, seed, progeny . . . food or feed product . . ."; "DNA, transgenic plant (rice, wheat . . . vegetables as carrot, bean, cabbage . . . berries and fruits as strawberry, grape, banana . . . sorghum, tobacco . . . "; "DNA from rice, polypeptide, transformed plant (cereal, potato, wheat, rice, corn, oat, barley, rye, dicot), producing a product (seed, fruit, vegetable, progeny, plant, seed . . .) . . ."; "DNA from rice, plant which is rice, wheat, corn, potato, bean, vegetables, fruit trees, pepper, apple, sorghum . . ."; "DNA from rice, transgenic plant, progeny, seed, rice, wheat . . . vegetables, fruit trees, spices, berries . . . method of enhancing pathogen resistance (nematode, bacteria, fungus, virus, viroid)." As of this writing, the patent application is still pending.

If the prospect of a large corporation owning the patent rights to genes in all the world's flowering plants, as well as the patent for the process of photosynthesis, doesn't scare you, you may need to have someone take your pulse to make sure you are still among the living. Or you could try rereading the previous section about Percy Schmeiser, and then sit down and take notes while watching a science fiction movie about aliens who are aiming for world domination.

You can help fight back by buying food that does not contain genetically modified ingredients, by planting non–genetically modified vegetable seeds, and by supporting the Seed Savers Exchange, which is an organization that is preserving thousands of heirloom and non–genetically modified seeds.

A few sources for non–genetically modified seeds:

Seed Savers Exchange: www.seedsavers.org
Fedco Seeds: www.fedcoseeds.com
Territorial Seed Company: www.territorialseed.com
Seeds of Change: www.seedsofchange.com
Johnny's Selected Seeds: www.johnnyseeds.com

## COTTONSEED OIL

The National Cottonseed Products Association informs us: "Cotton has long been known as nature's unique food and fiber plant. It produces both food for man and feed for animals in addition to a highly versatile fiber for clothing, home furnishings, and industrial uses."

Using everything and wasting nothing is generally a good idea, but unfortunately, worldwide, more pesticides are sprayed on cotton than on any other crop. According to the Pesticide Action Network North America, more than 10 percent of the pesticides and nearly 25 percent of the insecticides used in the world each year are used on cotton crops. After the cotton fibers are extracted from the cotton bolls, the cottonseeds are cleaned and the oil is extracted. Every year, half a million tons of cottonseed oil go into salad dressings, baked goods, and snack crackers and chips. Three million tons of cottonseed cake are fed to beef and dairy cattle, along with enormous quantities of gin trash, which is the fuzz and contaminants left over after the cotton fiber has been cleaned.

The cotton industry claims that when the cottonseed oil is treated, all the pesticide residues are removed. Unfortunately, cottonseeds are toxic, whether or not the cotton plants were doused with pesticides. The stems, roots, and seeds of the cotton plant (scientific name, *Gossypium*) contain a highly toxic yellow pigment called gossypol, which helps protect the plants from the predations of herbivorous animals and insects. The toxin is most highly concentrated in the seeds.

In 1957, health care workers in Jiansu Province, China, noticed a high incidence of childlessness in families in the area. Crude cottonseed oil was commonly used as a cooking oil in the province, and upon further investigation, it became apparent that men who consumed the largest quantities of cottonseed oil were sterile. In 1971, a Chinese research team showed that male rats that were fed gossypol were rendered temporarily infertile.

Though the cottonseed oil that is so ubiquitous in the American diet is refined to remove the gossypol, the cottonseed meal that is commonly used as a cheap source of protein for farm animals is not. The cottonseed meal contains gossypol, which if ingested in sufficient quantities can affect the health of the animals.

D. Nagalakshmi, A. K. Sharma, and V. R. B. Sastry, of the Indian Veterinary Research Institute in Uttar Pradesh, India, fed rations that contained 40 percent cottonseed meal to three- to four-month-old lambs for 180 days. The researchers studied the tissues of the sacrificial lambs and found that the males' testes were devoid of sperm and sperm-producing cells, and the seminiferous tubules were collapsed.

J. Velasquez-Pereira, et al., tested the long-term effects of cottonseed meal in the diets of twenty-four Holstein bulls that were approximately six months old when the study began. For the next ten months the bulls were fed either soybean meal with vitamin supplements, or cottonseed meal with vitamin supplements. The cottonseed-fed bulls had abnormally leaky red blood cells, and high concentrations of gossypol had built up in their livers, hearts, and testes. Gossypol is known to cause edema; liver, thyroid, and heart damage; hemorrhage; and reproductive disorders and birth defects in many animal species.

A 1996 USDA study showed a buildup of gossypol in the livers, hearts, muscle, and spleens of lambs who had been fed cottonseed meal.

If you are what you eat, do you really want to eat gossypol-enhanced meat from animals who have been fed cotton trash?

## OF COMPLICATIONS AND COWS

In 1943, the U.S. Second Circuit Court commented on the complexities of the governmental regulations of dairy products: "The milk problem is exquisitely complicated. The city dweller or poet who regards the cow as a symbol of bucolic serenity is indeed naive. . . . The milk problem is so vast that to fully comprehend it would require an almost universal knowledge ranging from geology, biology, chemistry and medicine to the niceties of the legislative, judicial and administrative processes of government. . . ."

Things have only gotten more complicated since then. Now, in order to understand dairy regulations, one also needs a good grasp of genetic engineering and biotechnology patent laws.

Cows produce more milk in the spring and summer, when their calves are young; milk production drops as the calves mature. Consequently, dairy herds that are large enough to meet the demand for milk in the cooler months produce a surplus during warmer weather. The U.S. government has been buying surplus milk from farmers for many decades in order to help stabilize dairy prices and help the farmers stay in business. Despite the fact that American cows were already producing an excess of milk, in the 1990s Monsanto developed and then marketed a genetically recombined hormone that, when injected into a cow, would make her produce 10 to 20 percent more milk. This artificial growth hormone is known as recombinant Bovine Growth Hormone (rBGH), or recombinant Bovine Somatrophin (rBST), and is sold to dairy farmers under the brand name Posilac. The Food and Drug Administration approved the product in 1993, and both the FDA and Monsanto claim that there is no measurable difference between milk produced naturally by cows and milk produced by cows that are juiced up with rBGH. This is the basis for the numerous lawsuits that Monsanto has initiated against dairy farmers who have labeled their naturally produced milk as "rBGH free." In a 2007 letter to the Federal Trade Commission (FTC), Monsanto stated that the "deceptive advertising and labeling practices" of milk producers and processors misleads consumers "by falsely claiming that there are health and safety risks associated with milk from rBST-supplemented cows."

In October 2007, the State of Pennsylvania sent warnings to nineteen dairies informing them that "their labels are false or misleading and need to be changed." Here are a few examples of the offending language: "Our farmers' pledge: no artificial growth hormones," "Free of artificial growth hormones," and "From cows not treated with the growth hormone rBST." These labels were considered so inflammatory that the Pennsylvania Department of Agriculture (PDA) outlawed any labeling that identified a milk product as having been produced without the use of synthetic hormones. The law was to go into effect in February 2008. The subsequent uproar from consumers all over the country convinced the PDA to reverse its decision in January 2008. But other bills restricting the use of "rBST-free" labels were introduced in state legislatures in New Jersey, Kansas, Utah, Indiana, and Missouri.

Cow's milk, like all other milk produced by female mammals, contains hormones, so Monsanto's claim that its product causes no measurable differences in the type or amount of hormones in the milk produced by treated cows may be technically true, but that does not necessarily mean that injecting dairy cows with hormones every two weeks is a safe and sane practice. A Vermont study showed that mastitis (infection of the udder) is seven times as common among cows that have been treated with rBGH, and the infection takes six times longer to treat than does mastitis that is not associated with rBGH. Another study showed that farmers often treat this recalcitrant mastitis with antibiotics that are not approved for use in dairy cattle, and yet another study showed that antibiotic-resistant bacteria were one-third more common in rBGH-treated cattle than in untreated cows.

A technical manual distributed to veterinarians by Monsanto states that when rBST-treated cows get mastitis, the infection is 62 percent more likely to be caused by *Staphylococcus aureus*. And apparently staphylococcus really likes antibiotics in milk. A 1993 study showed that *S. aureus* developed resistance to antibiotics 600 percent faster when swimming in milk that contained residue from an antibiotic. When it was immersed in milk that contained residues from three different antibiotics, *S. aureus* evolved antibiotic-resistance 2,700 percent faster.

In 2007, researchers at the Central Veterinary Institute in Budapest, Hungary, isolated methicillin-resistant *Staphylococcus aureus* (MRSA) from cows that had mastitis, and collected samples of the same strain of bacteria from the cows' caretaker. Whether or not we drink milk, an increase in the population of drug-resistant pathogens endangers all of us.

## WHEN THE DAIRY DOOR CLOSES, ANOTHER DOOR OPENS

Cows injected with rBGH require higher protein feed. The artificially sped-up cows live faster and burn out several years sooner than normal. But when one phase of a dairy cow's useful life has ended, another has just begun. According to Ted C. Perry, the beef cattle extension associate at Cornell's College of Agriculture and Life Science in New York, "Cull cows are a huge resource of hamburger in this country, where 50 percent of the beef we consume is hamburger." He added that "most of the 10.5 million pounds of hamburger eaten by New Yorkers each year comes from former dairy cows."

Milk that contains rBGH/rBST has been banned in the European Union, Canada, Australia, New Zealand, Japan, and most other industrialized countries, and the hormone has been quite unpopular with American consumers, who have been speaking loudly, repeatedly, and incessantly ever since rBGH milk hit the market. American companies are finally responding: Within the last year, Chipotle, Starbucks, Tillamook, and Kroger announced that they will no longer buy or sell products containing rBGH milk, and Wal-Mart and Safeway, Inc., have changed their store brands to non-rBGH milk.

Finally, in August 2008, Monsanto announced that it planned to sell the division that manufactures rBGH. The company insisted that there is nothing wrong with the product and denied that pressure from consumers influenced their decision. The pharmaceutical giant Eli Lilly bought the division for more than $300 million, and continues to push the states to pass legislation that would ban labels that say "rBGH free."

Perhaps the pharmaceutical industry should work on drugs that would make consumers cease to care whether or not their food supply is safe and nutritious.

## KEEPING OUR STRENGTH UP

But what, the skeptics ask, about the problem of global hunger? Isn't it necessary to use synthetic fertilizers, hormones, pesticides, and herbicides in order to feed an increasingly hungry world? Isn't organic food just for elitists and worrywarts? Researchers from the University of Michigan studied the relationship between organic farming and crop yields, and concluded that in developed countries, the crop yields from organic and conventional farms were almost equal, while in developing countries, food production would double or even triple if the farmers all switched to organic methods. In a study published in the July 4, 2007, issue of *Renewable Agriculture and Food Systems*, Professor Ivette Perfecto and her colleagues found that organic farming could produce harvests that were equal to or greater than those produced by conventional agricultural methods, and that these organic harvests could be achieved without putting additional cropland into production by using readily available quantities of organic fertilizers. According to Perfecto, organic farming is important because conventional agriculture, with its mechanized tillage, synthetic fertilizers, and chemical poisons, causes soil erosion, emits greenhouse gases, and reduces biodiversity. As if that were not enough, the fertilizer- and chemical-runoff from conventional farms is the chief cause of low-oxygen dead zones in the oceans. Perfecto called the notion that people would go hungry if all farming went organic "ridiculous" and added, "Corporate interest in agriculture and the way agriculture research has been conducted in land grant institutions, with a lot of influence by the chemical companies and pesticide companies as well as fertilizer companies—all have been playing an important role in convincing the public that you need to have these inputs to produce food."

The choice between synthetic and organic food may become moot one of these days. Petroleum prices are skyrocketing, and the cost of petroleum-based agrochemicals is rising right along with them. Many conventional farmers, who considered organic fertilizers too expensive in 2007, became instant converts in 2008 when natural fertilizers were, for the first time, far cheaper than the petroleum-based variety.

And as fertilizer prices rise, hog manure—a substance that not long ago was treated with great disdain—has become a hot commodity. Unwanted hog manure languishing in a manure lagoon is indeed an environmental nightmare, but hog manure spread judiciously in a field is an environmentally friendly fertilizer. Now farmers in Iowa are cutting deals with hog producers to build hog barns on the edges of their corn and soybean fields.

## COUCH TATERS

In the spring of 2008, American officials at the highest level of government (who shall remain nameless) made statements blaming India's rising prosperity for the recent precipitate rise in global food prices. Pradeep S. Mehta, secretary-general of the Center for International Trade, Economics, and the Environment in Jaipur, India, promptly retorted that the global food shortage has clearly been created by Americans, who consume far more calories than does the typical Indian citizen, and added that if Americans slimmed down to the weight of middle-class Indians, "many hungry people in sub-Saharan Africa would find food on their plates."

Mr. Mehta may have a point. According to United Nations data, each American eats an average of 3,770 calories every day, which is the highest caloric intake in the world, while the average Indian takes in 2,440 calories per day. It takes approximately 18 calories per pound to maintain the weight of a very active person, 15 calories per pound to maintain the weight of a moderately active person, and 13 calories per pound to maintain the weight of a sedentary person. Thus, the 3,770-calorie American diet is enough to maintain the weight of a very active 209-pound person, a moderately active 251-pound person, or a 290-pound couch potato. The 2,440-calorie Indian diet is enough to maintain the weight of a very active 136-pound person, a moderately active 163-pound person, or a 188-pound couch samosa. Notice that the American couch potato outweighs his Indian counterpart by more than 100 pounds. Lugging that extra weight around requires extra fuel, and growing the food to maintain that excess avoirdupois requires extra fuel, fertilizer, and land.

Unfortunately, many of the excess calories in the American diet are from fast food and junk foods. Even if we could, we shouldn't export our excess fast-food burgers, fries, and shakes to starving people in Third World countries. Starving people need to be given the wherewithal to produce their own food using their own local resources.

Heifer International is a nonprofit organization that provides livestock and agricultural training to families around the world. The simple gift of a cow, a goat, or a pig can lift an entire family out of poverty. Since 1944, Heifer International has helped 9.2 million families in 125 countries (www.heifer.org).

## BETTER FOR YOU, BETTER FOR THE ENVIRONMENT

A recent study by the Union of Concerned Scientists showed that most grass-fed beef contains less fat per serving than does corn-fed beef, and the fat in the grass-fed beef contains higher percentages of omega-3 fatty acids, which may help reduce the risk of heart disease.

In 2007, Cornell researchers published a study in the journal *Renewable Agriculture and Food Systems* in which they examined the land requirements of human diets. The researchers compared forty-two different diets made up of foods that could be grown in New York State. All the diets supplied the same number of calories, though the different diets included varying amounts of meat, ranging from none to 13.4 ounces daily. The diets also contained different percentages of fat, ranging from 20 to 40 percent of the total caloric content of the diet.

Chris Peters, Ph.D., the lead author of the study, stated: "A person following a low-fat vegetarian diet, for example, will need less than half (0.44) an acre per person per year to produce their food. . . . A high-fat diet with a lot of meat, on the other hand, needs 2.11 acres."

Dr. Peters stated: "Surprisingly, however, a vegetarian diet is not necessarily the most efficient in terms of land use." The reason for this apparent contradiction is that fruits, vegetables, and grains require high-quality cropland. Meat and dairy products can be produced on lower-quality land that is unsuitable for growing field crops, but can support pasture and hayfields. This lower-quality pastureland is more widely available than prime agricultural land, and in order to maintain soil fertility, most field crops need to be planted in a rotation with perennial crops such as pasture and hay. Dr. Peters's conclusion was: "It appears that while meat increases land-use requirements, diets including modest amounts of meat can feed more people than some higher fat vegetarian diets."

Note: Free-range bison use even fewer resources than do free-range cattle. Many ranchers and farmers have already quit raising cattle and begun raising bison.

## COWS IN BERKELEY?

The safest food will always be that which you either grow yourself or is produced by people you know. We are what we eat; we are also what our food eats.

Though the idea of cows within city limits now strikes most of us as strange, dairy cows were once common in urban areas. Before cars became common, the horses that worked in the city were stabled in the city, so small dairies that contained a cow or two probably seemed quite natural. If you look closely, you will find that some older homes have free-standing garages whose doors look suspiciously like barn doors. Unfortunately, it does not seem as if large livestock will be reappearing in urban centers anytime soon.

When I was a teenager, I often went on weekend overnight hikes into the beautiful hills of the nearby dairy country. All day long the resident bovines placidly munched their way across steep hillsides on trails so astonishingly narrow and treacherous that I had trouble traversing them in my hiking boots. When evening came the cows would wind their way home to the milking barn. These cows were living, breathing examples of why human beings keep livestock: Farm animals are capable of extracting food value from substances that humans cannot eat, and they can accomplish this in areas where humans cannot plant crops.

In 2008, the U.S. Department of Agriculture approved a rule that would allow a "USDA Process Verified Grass Fed" label on beef from cattle that were on pasture during the growing season. This label means that an inspector has verified that the cattle in question are indeed being pastured on grass.

## "GREEN" EGGS AND HAM

Chickens and pigs are omnivores that enjoy worldwide popularity because they happily ingest leftovers, scraps, peels, and other food waste that is not suitable for human consumption. These miraculous creatures then turn waste into food. Though most municipalities frown upon urban swine-keeping, one need not move to the country in order to enjoy freshly laid eggs produced by happy hens. Many municipalities, including San Francisco and Oakland, California; New York City; Houston; Chicago; Seattle; and Portland, Oregon, allow residents to keep laying hens, and people in many other cities keep laying flocks despite their illegality. Many of these urban flocks are large enough to produce marketable quantities of eggs.

## SUCKING EGGS

Irma Rombauer's *The Joy of Cooking* is justly famous because it is so impressively all-inclusive. (If you need to know how to prepare bracken fern fronds, or how to clean and cook rabbit, muskrat, woodchuck, beaver, peccary, wild boar, venison, fish, lobster, live shellfish, abalone, snapping turtles, or escargot, Mrs. Rombauer is your woman.) Yet, though my ancient, frontless-and-backless edition of *The Joy of Cooking* contains quite a few recipes for delicacies that contain raw eggs, it sounds nary a warning about lurking microbial dangers. Mrs. Rombauer did not mention the dangers of ingesting raw eggs because when she wrote the book in 1931, raw eggs were still perfectly safe to eat; people had been eating them for millennia.

Beginning in the 1960s, sporadic epidemics of salmonella poisoning struck people who had eaten raw or undercooked eggs. At first, researchers believed that the contamination was on the outside of the eggshells, and the USDA instituted strict new egg-washing regulations for commercial egg producers. These measures worked for a while, but then the salmonella epidemics started up again. In the 1980s, researchers did some detective work and determined that salmonella outbreaks going back to at least 1973 had been caused by bacteria that had been living inside clean, uncracked, Grade A eggs. Experiments at the University of Pennsylvania proved that the bacteria were lodged in the egg yolks rather than in the egg whites. The infected eggs were being laid by infected hens. For millennia, raw eggs had been safe for humans to eat, but in the twentieth century, the raw egg mutated into an object of fear and loathing.

Further research suggested that the culprit was indoor, factory-style egg and poultry production that segregated baby chicks from older chickens and their droppings. If baby chicks are not exposed to the beneficial bacteria that inhabit the guts of older chickens, their guts tend to be colonized by dangerous bacteria such as *Salmonella enteritidis*, campylobacter, listeria, and the deadly *E. Coli* O157:H7. These bacteria don't seem to bother the birds, but when infected chicks grow up into laying hens, they lay infected eggs; and infected roasters or broilers must be cooked until they are very well done.

The problem of pathogenic chickens can be dealt with in a couple of different ways:

- Spray the baby chicks with a commercially formulated blend of beneficial bacteria that normally inhabit the intestines of adult chickens. (Beneficial microbes that protect their host against disease are called probiotics.) The chicks ingest the bacteria when they preen their fuzz, and the beneficial bacteria quickly colonize their intestines and outcompete the dangerous bacteria.
- Raise chickens the old-fashioned way: in a coop with enough room for them to walk around in, and allow them outside to play as often as possible.

 I prefer the second alternative, and have kept a small flock of laying hens for several years now. I can see them from the window over my kitchen sink, and find them endlessly amusing.

Eggs from my free-range hens, and from any other hens that are allowed to roam around and scratch in the dirt regularly, are generally perfectly safe to eat raw.

## THIS WILL CURL THEIR TAILS

Probiotic bacteria are also good for pigs. A group of researchers led by Pat G. Casey of University College, Cork, Ireland, published a paper in the March 2007 issue of *Applied and Environmental Microbiology* in which they described the effects of probiotic food on fifteen weanling piglets.

The researchers gave the groups of piglets a daily dose of either plain milk or milk that contained a mixture of five probiotic strains of lactobacillus commonly found in fermented milk products such as yogurt or kefir. After six days of this regimen, all the piglets were given a dose of live, pathogenic salmonella bacteria. The subjects' health was monitored for twenty-three days after they were infected. The researchers found that "Animals treated with probiotics showed reduced incidence, severity, and duration of diarrhea. These animals also gained weight at a greater rate than control pigs administered skim milk." The probiotic piglets were also apparently producing probiotic manure, because two weeks after they were infected, they were shedding far less salmonella bacteria than were the nonprobiotic piglets.

Salmonella infection is a major cause of gastroenteritis in humans. Using probiotics to reduce the amount of salmonella being shed by livestock into the environment would be a very good thing.

## CULTIVATING USEFUL FRIENDS

Scientists tell us that the average human gut contains about one hundred different species of bacteria, including probiotic bacteria that help us digest our food and synthesize some B vitamins and vitamin K. The average human being is made up of ten trillion human cells, but the average human's intestinal tract contains one hundred trillion bacteria. The entire length of the intestine is lined with a layer of bacteria that can be up to one inch thick; these beneficial bacteria vigorously hold and defend their territory against invading pathogenic bacteria and yeasts, and encourage their host's immune system to produce antibodies against dangerous intruders. I need as many friends as I can get, and toward that end, I consume as many probiotic foods as I can swallow. My gut is awash in yogurt, kefir, kimchi, dill pickles, salami, and sauerkraut.

## KIMCHI

Kimchi, sometimes called the national food of Korea, is a hot, spicy, pickled mélange of Chinese cabbage and other ingredients such as peppers, onion, garlic, radishes, and ginger. Kimchi is rich in probiotic bacteria, including lactobacillus, streptococcus, pediococcus, and leuconostoc.

A study headed by Kun-Young Park of Pusan National University, Pusan, Korea, published in the October 2003 issue of *Journal of Medicinal Food*, demonstrated that kimchi inhibits the growth of cancer cells.

In 2003, when thousands of people in Asia contracted SARS (severe acute respiratory syndrome), setting off a worldwide panic, kimchi consumption increased dramatically in Korea, because the people believed that eating kimchi could help protect them from the disease. They may have been right. In 2005, scientists at Seoul National University announced that they had fed kimchi extract to thirteen chickens that had been infected with bird flu, and a week later, eleven of the birds had started to recover.

Though the researchers admitted that they had no idea how or why the kimchi might have cured the birds, their study sparked a worldwide boom in the sales of kimchi and sauerkraut, the German version of kimchi. Ryan Downs, the owner and general manager of Great Lakes Kraut Co., which has sauerkraut factories in Wisconsin and New York, told a reporter, "Unlike the government, we've got the preventative, and 115,000 tons of it in Wisconsin alone. . . . We're ready to help keep the world healthy."

Researchers at the University of New Mexico compared the incidence of breast cancer in Polish women and in Polish-born U.S. residents. The women who had eaten the most cabbage and/or sauerkraut during adolescence had the lowest risk of breast cancer. Women who had eaten 1.5 or fewer servings of cabbage or sauerkraut per week during adolescence were 74 percent more likely to get breast cancer than were those who had grown up eating four or more servings of kraut or cabbage per week.

## KEFIR, THE PROBIOTIC CHAMPION

Kefir, as I've mentioned, is a fermented milk product that is very healing when applied to the outside of the body. This beverage is even more salubrious when applied to the inside of the body. Kefir grains are so lively and complicated that the kefir they produce is difficult to standardize. Consequently, most commercial "kefir" is not made the traditional way, from kefir grains, but rather from a mixture of some, but not all, of the bacteria found in kefir grains. This standardized beverage is not as microbially complex as traditional kefir.

If you are lucky enough to acquire live kefir grains, making kefir is quite easy: Put the kefir grains and some milk in a glass or plastic container. Cover the container with a plastic lid (metal may react with the kefir, so metal lids and utensils are not recommended). Allow the container to sit at room temperature for twenty-four to forty-eight hours, until the milk coagulates. Remove the kefir grains and put them into another container with some milk. The finished kefir, sans grains, can be refrigerated and then drunk. Homemade kefir is sour, slightly fizzy, and very slightly alcoholic. Some connoisseurs refer to kefir as "the champagne of dairy products."

There is reason to believe that kefir is conducive to health, because the kefir-drinking and yogurt-eating people of the Caucasus and Azerbaijan are famous for their longevity. The Azerbaijanis are reported to have approximately five centenarians per ten thousand inhabitants. The latest U.S. census tells us that fewer than two out of every ten thousand Americans live to be one hundred.

Researchers have pitted kefir against a wide variety of maladies that they have inflicted on laboratory animals:

- A 2001 study conducted by Karine Thoreux and Douglas Lees Schmucker showed that feeding kefir to rats who had been exposed to cholera helped the animals fight off the disease more successfully than did rats who had not been fed kefir.
- A study conducted at the Natural Medicine Research Center in Korea demonstrated that feeding kefir to specially bred asthmatic laboratory mice made the mice less likely to have asthma attacks when they were exposed to allergens.
- Another mouse asthma study, conducted at the Medical University Children's Hospital in Warsaw, Poland, in 2007, demonstrated that feeding probiotic milk-fermenting bacteria to mice every other day from the time they were born until they were eight weeks old prevented them from developing the mouse version of asthma that they had been bred to demonstrate.
- Argentine researchers demonstrated that several strains of kefir bacteria prevent salmonella bacteria from sticking to and invading skin cells. (Perhaps we should eat our tomatoes with a kefir-based salad dressing.)

• Several studies have shown that many of the bacteria found in kefir can help make food safer by binding to chemical mutagens that are commonly found in food. (Mutagens are substances that can induce permanent genetic changes, which can cause birth defects, miscarriages, or cancer.)

Scientists have identified more than two dozen species of beneficial bacteria and a dozen species of helpful yeasts in kefir and kefir grains. In contrast, only about half a dozen different species of bacteria and zero fungi are used to culture yogurt.

## YOU EAT WHAT YOU ARE

If you are not squeamish, and you like to eat more than your fair share of certain delicacies, you might try sharing the following information with some of your more finicky friends.

The sebaceous glands in the skin secrete sebum, a fatty material that helps keep hair and skin soft, pliable, and relatively waterproof. Propionibacteria live inside the sebaceous glands of adults and adolescents, where they busily produce carbon dioxide and stinky propionic acid as metabolic waste products. Propionibacteria are also responsible for creating the holes and the flavor of Swiss and other "large eye" cheeses.

Brevibacteria live between our toes, happily feeding on dead skin. As these bacteria feed, they produce the charming smell of dirty socks and dirty feet. They are also essential in the production of soft, stinky cheeses such as Limburger, Liederkrantz, Bel Paese, and Muenster. The odor of these cheeses is so distinctive that the French surrealist poet Leon-Paul Fargue (1876–1947) wrote, *"Le camembert, ce fromage qui fleure les pieds du bon Dieu"* (Camembert, this cheese that smells of the feet of the good God).

Various species of lactobacilli are part of the normal intestinal, vaginal, oral, and urethral flora of healthy human beings. They are also found in yogurt, kefir, some cheeses, sourdough starter, and other fermented foods such as kimchi, real dill pickles, and sauerkraut. You are what you eat, and apparently, if you want to remain healthy, you eat what you are.

## LEAVE ALL THE DOORS AND WINDOWS OPEN

There are five major types of beer, four of which—lagers, porters, stouts, and most ales—are brewed under nearly sterile conditions meant to exclude bacteria from the festivities. Hops, the flower bracts of a bitter herb that has antimicrobial properties, are added to these yeast-only beers in order to add flavor and to help fend off invading bacteria.

Belgian brewers have an entirely different approach to beer brewing. Rather than trying to exclude bacteria from the brewing process, they welcome them in. Belgian lambic beers, wheat beers, and some ales are full of complex flavors due to the complexity of the bacterial community that helped make them. No yeast is added to the wort (the grain mash from which beer is brewed), but the windows and sometimes even the roofs of traditional Belgian breweries are kept open so that native bacteria can fall into the brewing vats. Cobwebs and dust adorn the walls, and well-aged barrels are used to store the beer while complex flavors develop. (As soon as I read about lambic beers, I had to try one. How could anyone possibly resist a product that is made with the help of dust and cobwebs?)

The flavors of aged French cheeses are also dependent upon native bacteria. French cheese is aged in cheese caves, every one of which harbors a unique population of molds and bacteria. The indigenous bacteria of each cave produce cheese with a distinctive flavor. It makes me hungry just thinking about it.

## A LOAF OF BREAD, A HUNK OF CHEESE, AND THOU?

Roquefort cheese is produced in the village of Roquefort-sur-Soulzon, in a cave-riddled region of France. Legend has it that a young shepherd, in pursuit of a shepherdess, left his lunch of bread and cheese in one of the limestone caves and didn't return for a year. In the meantime, the bread had turned moldy and had infected the cheese. The moldy bread was completely inedible, but the blue-streaked cheese was delicious.

Roquefort cheese is still made the same way: large, specially baked loaves of rye bread are allowed to mold, and are then used to inoculate the newly made cheese with *Penicillium roqueforti*. The cheese is then put in the limestone cave and allowed to soak up the atmosphere until it comes of age.

If you are interested in learning more about the everyday interactions between humans and bacteria, I recommend Betsey Dexter Dyer's amusing, useful, and informative tome *A Field Guide to Bacteria* (Cornell University Press, 2003).

## DRINKING LIKE A BARBARIAN—WATERED TO DEATH

There has never been a single documented case of a modern athlete dying of exercise-induced dehydration. Despite this fact, we have just suffered through approximately a decade of widespread dehydration neurosis that was largely promulgated by the bottled-water and sports-drink industries. Note: Dehydration and heatstroke are not the same thing.

Heatstroke occurs when the body's ability to cool itself is inadequate for the heat it is encountering, and the brain overheats. Humans are sweat-cooled creatures. When sweat evaporates from the surface of the skin, it carries away excess body heat. Both high humidity and excess clothing prevent sweat from evaporating.

The first marathoner died after he completed his run from Marathon to Athens in 491 B.C., but he had fought in a battle before he embarked.

Though there has never been a documented case of a modern marathoner dying of dehydration, between 1997 and 2005 there were eight documented cases of marathoners and army recruits dying of overhydration (the scientific term is hyponatremia, meaning low blood sodium). Nonelite runners who are drinking a cup of water every mile, as they have been encouraged to do, have been sloshing slowly along until they become nauseated, groggy, and incoherent, and then collapse. These symptoms occur because their blood is so excessively diluted that their soggy, swollen brains are pressing against their skulls, and some victims are even frothing pink at the mouth because of pulmonary edema (soggy lungs). Some have died on the spot; others have lapsed into comas and died in the hospital. Luckier ones have been successfully treated with intravenous salt solution, which pulls water out of their swollen brain cells, thus saving their lives.

Hyponatremia is an entirely preventable illness: Just drink when you're thirsty and stop when your thirst is slaked—you are not a camel crossing the Sahara Desert, you're a human being. If you have sweated quite heavily and feel really dried out after a workout, you might want to consider drinking either salty vegetable juice, some salty broth, or some milk, because in this case, clear liquids, even "sports drinks," do not contain enough electrolytes to prevent hyponatremia.

## HEAT SICK

On October 7, 2007, the Chicago Marathon was run under the hottest, most humid conditions in its thirty-year history. The temperature reached 88 degrees F. and the humidity was brutal. Hundreds of runners were treated for heat-related illnesses. One runner collapsed and died in the nineteenth mile of the race. Three and a half hours after it began, officials stopped the race, more than an hour after the fastest runners had crossed the finish line.

Forty-five thousand runners were registered for the race, but 9,133 of them did not show up. Some of these no-shows may have had some previous experience with heat.

If it's so hot that just breathing is making you sweat, it's probably too hot to exercise outside in the sun. Defying the elements will get you nowhere fast (except, perhaps, to the hospital). Noël Coward wrote a song about that kind of thing: "Mad dogs and Englishmen go out in the midday sun."

If it's really, really hot, pretend you're a wild animal and retreat to the modern equivalent of a nice, cool cave.

Heatstroke is always terribly dangerous, but healthy adults who have access to potable liquids are extremely unlikely to die of or even be made seriously ill by dehydration. Serious dehydration, in which the blood becomes dangerously concentrated, is almost always caused by disease. In fact, dehydration caused by diarrheal disease is the leading cause of death in infants and children worldwide.

If you are really worried about dehydration, rather than purchasing sports drinks, why not send the money to Save the Children, UNICEF, or another organization that works to improve children's health?

## CITY TREK

When you are trekking across the urban wilderness, you can be fairly confident that there will be drinking water available at your destination—that's the wonderful thing about civilization! But that may change as our planet heats up. I opened the paper on the morning of November 13, 2007, and learned that Governor Sonny Perdue of Georgia had resorted to rain prayers on the previous day in order to encourage God to make it rain. (The southern half of the United States was in the throes of a historic drought.)

If you can't drink water directly out of a public water fountain, do the environment a favor and drink out of a real water glass or a reusable metal or ceramic mug. If you like to carry your water with you, I suggest that you invest in a stainless-steel water bottle; it will not leach chemicals into your lovely, inexpensive tap water.

Not long ago I was at the checkout counter at the hardware store, and I idly began to read the hyperbolic copy on a sugar-free soft drink carton, on which the company extolled the taste, the lack of calories, and the fact that its product contains water. Fancy that! A beverage that contains water! What will they think of next? (For the record, urine contains the same percentage of water as does this company's product, so it could hydrate you, too.)

Some enlightening research was done recently on consumer preferences in soft drinks. Read Montague, of the Baylor College of Medicine in Houston, Texas, put volunteers into MRI machines in order to scan their brains while they were enjoying a drop of two well-known soft drink brands (literally a drop—people are lying down in MRI machines, so a big swig of liquid would make them choke). I will refer to these soft drinks as "Pop C" and "Pop P," so I don't get sued. Montague found that when the recumbent pop-tasters weren't told which brand they were sampling, the way the pleasure and reward centers of their brains lit up indicated that they preferred Pop P. When they were told which pop they were tasting, the parts of their brains that govern thought and memory lit up, indicating that they preferred Pop C.

It ain't the taste. It's the advertising.

 Frustrate a giant corporation. Drink tap water.

## OBJETS D'ART

Once upon a time, a few decades ago, I was a young art student eager to learn all I could about the grand endeavor of making Art. One fine weekend, one of my art classes took a field trip to the Oakland Museum. I felt it was my duty to gaze carefully and thoughtfully upon all the works of art, for they were obviously worthy, since they were in a museum. Sometimes this task became difficult and worrisome, especially in the "Bay Area Funk" room, which was full of sculptures so very whimsical and free-spirited that they looked as if they might fall apart at any moment. Because I was an Earnest Young Art Student, I gazed hard upon these ramshackle constructions, striving to understand their worthiness. After making the circuit of the room, I suddenly came upon a wonder! A well-made piece! A piece made by an artist who actually understood construction and materials, and had wrought the sculpture with skill and precision! I stared at this marvel, a metal wall sculpture so perfectly crafted, its corners so true, its finish so clean and pure, its door so perfectly fitted that it was a pleasure to look upon: "Thank God! Someone who knew what he was doing!" It was several minutes before I realized that I was admiring the fuse box. I quickly looked around to check for witnesses. When I realized that no one was near, I trotted off to find some of my classmates so I could reenact the scene for them.

It's all in the advertising.

## LIQUID PLACEBOS

Studies conducted by Professor Dan Ariely of MIT showed that "energy drinks" were only effective at increasing athletic and problem-solving performance when the subjects of the study believed the drinks were expensive. When a sports drink was sold to the research subjects for $2.89 a bottle, it improved the subjects' performance. When the same drink was sold to the subjects for eighty-nine cents per bottle, it caused a drop in performance, both when compared to the same drink sold for $2.89 and when compared to no drink at all.

The snob factor doesn't apply only to sports drinks. Researchers at the Stanford Graduate School of Business and the California Institute of Technology studied the effects of wine on the pleasure centers of the brain, and published their findings in January 2008 in the *Proceedings of the National Academy of Sciences*. Student volunteers were treated to individualized wine-tasting sessions inside an MRI machine, where each solitary supine subject sipped small samples of cabernet sauvignon through a high-tech straw. The volunteers were told that the MRI would trace their brain activity during the tasting process, which was true. They were also told that each wine, as it was delivered, would be identified by price, and the prices were: $5, $10, $35, $45, and $90 per bottle; the price information, however, was intentionally misleading. The researchers administered two wines twice each: the $5 and $45 wines were actually both the same $5 wine, and the $10 and $90 wines were both the same $90 wine. The correctly labeled $35 wine was used as a control. The students were asked to focus on the flavor and how much they enjoyed each sample. Brain scans revealed that the tasters enjoyed the $5 wine nearly twice as much when they thought they were drinking a $45 wine; and the pleasure of drinking the $90 wine was cut in half when the tasters thought they were drinking a $10 wine. The reactions of the taste-sensory centers of the brain don't change when wines are relabeled, but when people believe they are drinking an expensive wine, there is a lot more excitement in the part of the brain that decides how good it tastes. The researchers also found that pretty labels, good reviews, and brand names can also enhance wine-induced pleasure.

In an unrelated and more upright study, Brian Wansink, a Cornell University marketing professor, discovered that research subjects ate 12 percent more food, and lingered ten minutes longer at the table, when they were drinking trendy "California" wine rather than humble "North Dakota" wine. Both were the same wine.

## CONNOISSEURS

Some people, when life hands them lemons, make lemonade. In 2002, when life provided northern Minnesota with enough tent caterpillars (colloquially known as army worms) to smother every poplar tree between Hinkley and the Canadian border, Ray Reigstad of Duluth made wine. The *Duluth News Tribune* heard about Chez Reigstad's 2002 vintage, and invited four oenophiles to a wine tasting to sample a locally made wine. The tasters included a liquor store owner, a wholesale wine distributor, a wine cellar worker, and a day care operator named Jane who belonged to a wine club.

The tasters were asked to rate the wine on a scale of one to ten, with ten being the highest and one being the lowest.

The liquor store owner commented: "White wine with a slight tint of amber. Very acceptable appearance. Aroma is light with essence of sweetness and flowers. Body is medium light and very smooth. It's semi-dry, similar to a sauvignon blanc or pinot grigio. A slight oak finish with a bit of acidity. The wine overall is very acceptable and would pair nicely with chicken, pasta or fish. Overall rating: 7."

The wine wholesaler said: "Pale golden. Aroma: (bouquet) Light citrus. Crisp and dry, similar to sauvignon blanc or white Bordeaux. Clean start and a unique finish. An interesting wine, dry and slightly acidic with very slight undertones of melon or berry. It could be served with poultry or fish. Very nice for a locally produced wine. Overall rating: 7."

The wine cellar employee said: "Pale, reminiscent of a pinot grigio. Aroma: (bouquet) Apple, apricot, pear and a hint of subtle oak. It has an understated front, with a crisp citron middle and a grassy, deceptively robust finish. Its alter ego is a New Zealand white. Would pair well with pasta and light creamy sauces. Overall rating: 7."

Jane said, for the record: "Light, a little watery looking. Aroma: (bouquet) Light, fruity aroma. Interesting flavor, earthy undertones. A different finish and taste that lingers. I am usually a red wine drinker and this does not have the same complexity that most reds have. Although there are some subtle flavors that I can't quite identify. Overall rating: 4." (Off the record she said: "I didn't like it!")

After they had sipped and rated the wine, the tasters were told that the alcoholic beverage was made from squished caterpillars, not grapes.

## MORAL OF THE STORIES

Before your company arrives, take the price tag off that bottle and slap on a sticker with a higher number. (You will get away with this subterfuge. Experiments conducted by Frédéric Brochet at the University of Bordeaux proved that without accurate color cues, wine connoisseurs could not taste the difference between white and red wine.) If the wine originally came in a square container, decant it into something glass and cylindrical before you serve it. If your wine came in a pretty bottle with a screw top, just remove the cap and its rings, then put a real cork in it. Many experiments have shown that no one can taste the difference between a wine that has been stoppered with a natural cork and the same wine that has been stoppered with a synthetic cork or a metal screw top. But according to all the evidence, natural corks do not protect wine from spoilage as well as do synthetic corks or screw-on caps. Above all, just drink what tastes good to you—regardless of price, packaging, or whether it is made from caterpillars or grapes.

## COOKING WITH WINE

It is probable that as long as there has been wine, people have been cooking with it. And according to recent research, cooking with wine doesn't just improve the flavor of the food, it can also fend off food poisoning.

Research conducted by Mendel Friedman, of the U.S. Department of Agriculture, and colleagues has shown that marinating food in wine killed *Escherichia coli* 0157:H7, *Salmonella enterica*, *Bacillus cereus*, and *Listeria monocytogenes*, all of which can cause food poisoning. The researchers tested the antimicrobial capabilities of marinades concocted of Chardonnay, pinot noir, or sherry, mixed with various herbs and spices. Marinades that contained garlic, oregano, thyme, cloves, cinnamon, or lemongrass were all found to be effective at killing pathogens; the essential oils from the herbs and spices dissolve in the alcohol and add to its antimicrobial properties. The researchers suggested that these formulations could also be used as antimicrobial rinses and sprays that could be used to disinfect fruit, vegetables, meat, and poultry, as well as nonfood items such as cutting boards.

Note: If you want to marinate your cutting board and countertops in order to disinfect them, you might want to leave the garlic out of the marinade, and unless you want to dye your countertops a lovely, deep rich pink, use white wine rather than red.

## EATING LIKE A BARBARIAN

### EMOTIONAL EATING

Religion and culture color our attitudes toward food and often induce us to disapprove of other people's eating habits, despite the fact that humans are omnivorous by nature and thus any organic material that we can safely swallow, digest, and metabolize is suitable as food.

### NOURISHMENT

Spending money on cheap, processed food that cannot maintain your health is no bargain. No matter how cheap a precooked or processed food may seem, you are still paying someone else to do that cooking or processing. If your budget is tight, buy good, wholesome, unprocessed food and then try not to waste it.

If there is anywhere at all that you can plant some herbs or vegetables, do it! Many communities have city-sponsored community garden programs that help low-income people grow their own food in community garden plots. Many of these urban gardeners are making the transition from gardener to farmer, and are growing enough fruits and vegetables to sell in farmers' markets, where their fresh, local produce commands premium prices.

Landless urban gardeners often look upward, toward their roofs. In fact, studies conducted by New York Sun Works indicate that there is enough rooftop acreage across the five boroughs to provide fresh roof-garden vegetables to the entire city of New York.

For more information on urban agriculture, try visiting these websites:

Alternative Farming Systems Information Center: www.nal.usda.gov/afsic

Sustainable Agriculture Network: www.sare.org

USDA Community Food Project Grants: www.reeusda.gov/crgam/cfp/community .htm

This program is one of the most progressive things that our government has done in a long time. It is intended to increase food security in communities, improve self-reliance, and encourage entrepreneurship. The grants range in size from $10,000 to $250,000. If you have big ideas that require money, this would be worth exploring.

Alternative Farming Systems Information Center, National Agricultural Library: www.nal.usda.gov/afsic

American Community Gardening Association: www.communitygarden.org

Atlanta Urban Gardening: www.attra.org

Baltimore Grows: www.povertysolutions.org

Center for Urban Ecology: www.nps.gov/cue/cueintro

Cities Feeding People: www.idre.ca/cfp

City Farmer, Canada's Office of Urban Agriculture: www.cityfarmer.org

Community Food Security Coalition: www.foodsecurity.org

Food First: www.foodfirst.org

Gardens/Mini-Farms Network: www.minifarms.com

Green Guerrillas, New York: ggnyc@interport.net

Heifer Project International: www.heifer.org

International Development Research Centre (IDRC)

International Food Policy Research Institute (IFPRI): www.ifpri.cgiar.org

San Francisco League of Urban Gardeners (SLUG): www.slug-sf.org

Sustainable Agriculture Network, National Agricultural Library: www.sare.org

Urban Agriculture News: www.urbanagriculture-news.com

## FREEGANS

Every bite of food that is wasted means that more food will have to be produced, and extra production uses up more resources.

Luckily for all of us and for the environment, there are organizations such as Second Harvest that gather discarded-though-edible food from producers and distributors and redistribute it to people who need it, and there are also "Freegans," freelance Dumpster divers who joyfully harvest food from the urban environment. Rather than looking down our noses at those who glean, we should be heartily thanking them for their beneficial effect on the environment.

For many years, my composting worms have dined on compostable organic fruits and vegetables from our local natural foods co-op. The co-op obligingly segregates usable food waste from its trash by putting its bags of compostable food waste into a designated compost container, so that people can pick up thirty-gallon bags of clean, overripe fruits, dented vegetables, and wilted greens to feed to their animals. Quite frequently there are perfectly edible ripe fruits and untarnished vegetables amid the botanical wreckage, and these hardy survivors often end up feeding my family rather than my composting worms. Produce managers tend to discard produce as soon as it ripens completely, but I can't bear to throw lovely, perfectly ripe organic pears, apples, eggplants, or fresh, crisp romaine lettuce directly to my worms; the worms can wait for my leftovers.

Note: I have written a small, useful booklet called *Laverme's Handbook of Indoor Worm Composting*, which contains almost everything I have learned about vermicomposting in the past two decades. It is available at www.greenmercantile.com and at www.lavermesworms.com.

For more information on Freeganism, go to freegan.info.

For more information on Second Harvest, go to secondharvest.org.

## FOOD SAFETY TIPS FOR SCROUNGERS

### Avoidance List

Avoid meat, seafood, eggs, dairy products, sprouts, cut melons, and unpasteurized cider and juice. These foods must be refrigerated in order to remain edible, while Dumpsters tend to be unrefrigerated.

Avoid salvaging any foods that have contacted raw meat or seafood. (When foraging, pay careful heed to the law of gravity, which ensures that any item that is directly beneath a leaking package of raw meat will become contaminated.)

Avoid food that someone else has already begun eating. You don't know where that stranger's mouth has been!

Avoid cooked grains, which when unrefrigerated make a wonderful culture medium for food-poisoning bacteria. Moldy soft flour-based foods such as bread, cookies, cakes, and bagels cannot be salvaged; the mold goes too deep. Moldy tomatoes cannot be safely salvaged either.

Avoid bulging or oozing cans. Botulism makes cans bulge. Botulism poisoning is frequently fatal.

Avoid any food that looks or smells bad. It's better to be safe than sorry. The rules of food safety apply to Dumpsters as well as to refrigerators.

Note: Home refrigerator experiments in which neglected food has changed its shape, color, texture, or smell, or has grown a fuzzy coat of mold, can be fun, but they cannot be eaten, not even by chickens or pigs. Spoiled food is fit only for the compost pile or the vermicomposting bin.

### Easy Pickings

 Shiny fruits and vegetables such as apples, pears, plums, citrus fruit, zucchini, squash, and bell peppers that have glossy, protective skins that are easily cleaned are good. A little bit of mold will be quite obvious on a smooth-skinned fruit, and if you can cleanly cut all the mold out, you can still eat the fruit. Vegetables such as cabbage, lettuce, and onions can be cleaned by removing the outer layers.

Spraying produce with distilled white vinegar and hydrogen peroxide will help disinfect it. (See chapter 3 for more information on disinfecting with these sprays.)

## ORTS AND ENDS

I would like to think that the contents of a person's stomach do not constitute an accurate gauge of the content of her character. I would like to believe this because for many, many years the backbone of most of our family dinners consisted of soup made from stock rendered down from the bony wreckage of that week's roast chicken, or made from turkey backs and necks that I had purchased for twenty-nine cents a pound.

Here is a lovely quote from George Eliot's book *Silas Marner*: "the rich ate and drank freely, accepting gout and apoplexy as things that ran mysteriously in respectable families, and the poor thought that the rich were entirely in the right of it to lead a jolly life; besides, their feasting caused a multiplication of orts, which were the heirlooms of the poor."

> ort (ôrt) *n: pl* orts (ôrts) . . . remnants of food, refuse. A morsel left at a meal; a fragment; refuse.
> —*Webster's New International,* 1927

Orts, like many other things that are undervalued, often have more character and flavor than their more demure and refined counterparts. In order to get the most out of orts, one just has to know how to treat them. I tend to cook with orts and leftovers because they're cheap, while my friend Jean exploits them for their flavor because she's a fantastic cook and knows that the choicest, most tender foods are not usually the most flavorful. Character and flavor often come from toughness and hard knocks.

Leftovers are actually handy-dandy, preassembled flavor modules that can be used to spice up, among other things, soups, stews, bread, casseroles, soufflés, omelettes, salads, pasta, rice, pancakes, and pies. Use your imagination or consult *The Joy of Cooking,* which contains hundreds of recipes that celebrate leftovers.

Any leftover food that you will not be eating within a day or two should be packed into a suitable freezer container, labeled, and frozen for future use.

## FROZEN FRUIT

Prices are lowest and fruit quality is highest when the fruit is in season. If you want to reduce your food costs during the winter, you may want to buy, grow, or harvest large quantities of fruit when it is in season, and then freeze it. Frozen fruit retains its flavor quite well, and it is certainly much more comfortable to stand in front of a hot stove while canning fruit, making jams and jellies, or baking pies when the weather is cold than during the hot, humid harvest season.

Frozen berries can be eaten as is, blended into smoothies, stirred into pancake batter, or used in baking. Overripe bananas are often sold quite cheaply and are delicious when frozen. Peel the bananas, wrap them in waxed paper, and put them in a freezer bag or container. Later, when you crave a delicious, sweet frozen treat, take a frozen banana out of the freezer and peel down the waxed paper. You can protect your hand from frostbite by wrapping the bottom of the banana in a clean cloth napkin.

Excess apples can be peeled and sliced, then frozen for later use in pies.

## STRETCHING A CHICKEN

On April 12, 2008, the Haitian government collapsed after more than a week of riots over rising food prices. There have also been food riots in Egypt, Yemen, Burkina Faso, Cameroon, Indonesia, Ivory Coast, Mauritania, Mozambique, and Senegal.

According to the U.S. Environmental Protection Agency (EPA), more than a quarter of America's food goes to waste, and it costs $1 billion annually to dispose of this wasted food. The least we can do is to avoid wasting the food that we have bought with our hard-earned dollars.

Those of you who have never needed to make a single chicken yield half a week's worth of dinners should thank your lucky stars. But if you should ever need to make food stretch farther, you might want to try some of the following techniques and recipes for stretching food.

These recipes require the following equipment:

Two six-quart stainless-steel stockpots. Avoid making soup in
    reactive pots such as aluminum, copper, brass, unenameled cast
    iron, or in pots with a nonstick coating that may contaminate
    your supper.
A metal colander. When put on top of the stockpot, the main body
    of the colander should hang down inside the stockpot, while
    the colander's handles rest securely on the stockpot's rim.
A stove.
A freezer.
Freezer bags or containers.
Metal tongs.
A metal ladle.
An electric Crock-Pot or slow cooker—optional, but recommended.

The fumes emitted by the nonstick coating on certain pots and pans have been known to kill caged birds. Studies conducted by the Environmental Working Group have shown that some overheated nonstick pans can emit fumes that contain chemicals that have been linked to cancer and birth defects. I would rather cook in a rusty old tin can than in a nonstick pan. The nontoxic choices for pots and pans include stainless steel, cast iron, tempered glass, and enameled cast iron.

The freezer is a soup maker's best friend. Almost any food that is not sweetened can be used in a soup. For instance, when you are preparing fresh vegetables, save the trimmings and put them in a large container in the freezer. Carrot peelings, potato skins, cabbage cores, wilted lettuce and other salad greens, trimmings from celery, broccoli, and cauliflower stems and leaves are all valuable additions to soup stock. (Note: Do not save green potato peelings or potato eyes! The green pigment is toxic.) If you are not planning to eat it the next day, an undressed, leftover salad can also be poured into your frozen container of soup vegetables.

Table scraps, leftover cooked foods, meat bones, and poultry carcasses can all be used to improve the flavor and nutritional qualities of a soup. If your dinner companions are not actually radioactive, it is unlikely that the leftovers on anyone's plate are more contaminated than the food was in its original state. Raw chickens are often contaminated with salmonella, but your dining companions probably aren't. Remember that the orts retrieved from your plates will be boiled in water for several hours. Pathogens will succumb.

Here's what to save and how to save it for brothmaking.

When you clean up after a carnivorous meal, the picked-clean carcass and bones can be put into a sturdy, one-gallon freezer bag and frozen. Other plate scrapings such as baked potato skins, rice, or the occasional green bean can also be put in the soup-makings bag—when the bag is full, it's time to make soup.

If you make a point of freezing any leftovers that you don't intend to eat within a day, you will quickly build up a useful stockpile of soup-making materials, and your food dollar will stretch farther than you ever thought possible. Cooked foods such as rice, potatoes, pasta, green beans, greens, squash, and almost any other food that someone has spent time and effort cooking and seasoning can be frozen and later added to your finished broth to make really delicious soups. Leftover bread can be used to thicken soups. But when you are freezing leftovers, detailed labeling is important, as is keeping highly seasoned foods segregated from each other. For instance, leftover lamb curry in a nice, strong chicken broth would make a delicious soup, and leftover eggplant parmesan added to chicken broth is lovely, but mixing them together might not be a good idea.

If you are desperately low on cash, and Dumpster diving is not your style, check out the meat section of your local supermarket or grocery store. Many stores sell packages of turkey backs and necks quite cheaply: The price for these humble parts has hovered between twenty-nine and sixty-nine cents a pound for the past twenty years.

After you've assembled all your orts, it's time to start cooking.

Put two pounds of rinsed turkey necks and backs and/or a gallon of meat or poultry bones in a large stockpot, cover with cold water, bring it to a boil on the stove, then turn down the heat and simmer it for a few hours. Fresh or frozen vegetable scraps and peelings can be simmered along with the bones.

> Do not salt the soup before it is completely finished, or it may become too salty as it cooks down. Salt should be the last thing that is added to a soup, broth, gravy, or sauce. But if you accidentally oversalt your soup, you can peel a raw potato and drop it into the simmering soup. As the potato cooks, it will soak up excess salt. When the potato is cooked through, remove it. If the soup is extremely salty, more than one potato may be necessary. (This method also works for salty sauces and stews.)

The broth is ready when it is opaque and the meat has lost all of its flavor. Set your metal colander into the top of your empty stockpot. Use metal tongs to remove the boiled bones from the stock. After you have removed all the bones from the stock, use the ladle to pour the stock through the colander in the empty stockpot. Once the stock has been strained into the new pot, you can begin to add soup fixings such as vegetables, rice, or pasta.

If you are going to use a Crock-Pot, now is the time to put a small amount of water in the bottom of the Crock-Pot and turn it on high. (One cannot safely add a hot liquid to a cold Crock-Pot; the heat stress can crack the ceramic crock.) Allow all the vegetables and other fixings to cook completely through before transferring the soup to the preheated Crock-Pot, where the soup can simmer safely all day without burning.

An alternate way to simmer the bones is to bring them to a boil in your stockpot, then transfer them to a Crock-Pot or slow cooker for long-term simmering. A broth can simmer safely for a day or two in a Crock-Pot.

The solids that were strained out of the broth can either be composted or put in a disposable bag and stored in the freezer until garbage day.

## JEWISH PENICILLIN

In the twelfth century A.D., the Jewish-Egyptian physician and philosopher Maimonides recommended chicken soup for "rectifying corrupted humors," which meant that it was a cure-all or panacea. Maimonides's recommendation was supposedly based on advice from classical Greek sources, and Jewish mothers have followed his prescription ever since.

Simmering poultry carcasses or meat bones for hours produces a delicious broth that will nourish you, and may also cure what ails you. Slowly simmered chicken soup contains substances such as dissolved cartilage from the bone knuckles and skin, collagen (gelatine), and chondroitin sulfate. Drinking homemade broth is certainly environmentally preferable to buying capsules of shark cartilage or shark-derived chondroitin in order to ease one's joint pain.

A tablespoon of vinegar or a cup of wine added to the cooking water at the beginning of the broth-making process will help draw more minerals out of the bones and will make the broth even more salubrious.

As to chicken soup versus the common cold: Barbara O. Rennard, Ronald F. Ertl, Gail L. Gossman, Richard A. Robbins, M.D., F.C.C.P., and Stephen I. Rennard, M.D., F.C.C.P., studied the anti-inflammatory properties of chicken soup, and their results were published in the journal *Chest* in 2000. The researchers hypothesized that most of the symptoms related to colds are caused by the body's inflammatory response to the cold virus. This response includes a migration of neutrophils (white blood cells) to the epithelial surface of the airways.

Following a traditional family recipe, the researchers simmered up a batch of classic chicken soup with matzoh balls, which was thereafter formally referred to as "Grandma's soup." Samples were taken from the soup pot before the chicken began to cook, when the water first began to boil, and after each new ingredient was added. These samples were allowed to cool and were then added to prepared neutrophils and allowed to incubate for half an hour. The researchers found that the chicken soup hindered the migration of the neutrophils. The stronger the chicken soup, the more it inhibited the neutrophils. The researchers admitted that it was unknown whether chicken soup would inhibit the inflammatory response in people with colds, but did state that since the active ingredient is water-soluble, it may be absorbable. They noted that the inhibitory effect was observed at dilutions as low as 1:200, which is "comparable to the dilution of a 350-mL 'average' bowl of soup eaten by a 70-kg person." They concluded that chicken soup could therefore have an anti-inflammatory effect in the human body.

## WILD GLEANING

Almost everywhere there are people, there are experts who gather wild edible plants, even in the middle of big metropolises. Many of these experts share their knowledge by teaching community education classes on gathering and preparing wild foods. If you are not already knowledgeable about plants, it is a good idea to learn from an expert before striking out on your own. Wild greens should never be harvested from contaminated soil or next to roadways because greens tend to accumulate heavy metals.

Many wild plants are not only more nutritious than their cultivated brethren, they also emerge earlier in the spring than most cultivated vegetables. Many of these plants are considered "weeds" by the uninitiated, but some of my favorite foods grow wild, including: lamb's-quarters (*Chenopodium album*)—a green, leafy plant that is delicious steamed, sautéed, or in soups and is related to beets, spinach, and Swiss chard; purslane (*Portulaca oleracea*)—a small, low-growing, fleshy-leafed plant with a slightly lemony tang that is good in salads and can be used as an okra substitute in gumbo; and last, but not least, stinging nettle (*Urtica dioica*), which has a meaty, brothy taste and contains impressive amounts of vitamins and minerals.

Every spring my family eagerly anticipates our first meal of steamed lamb's-quarters, which is delicious dipped in mayonnaise or melted butter. Lamb's-quarters also makes a delicious and nutritious addition to soups, so every growing season I harvest as much as I can and stow it in the freezer so I can add it to winter soups.

Nettles make such a valuable addition to our diet that I brought some plants home from a friend's farm about fifteen years ago, and transplanted them again when we moved to our country home. The secret to gathering nettles is to pick them while wearing rubber gloves or plastic bags on one's hands—the stinging hairs are far too delicate to sting through a plastic barrier. After the nettles are cooked, frozen, or dried, the sting disappears. I pick and dry or freeze many pounds of nettles each growing season so I can add nettles to my soups all winter long.

Weeds: If you can't beat 'em, eat 'em.

## ENTOMOPHAGY

 Inedibility often exists in the mind of the beholder: Your delicacy may be rejected by my culture or proscribed by my religion, and vice versa. Many Westerners happily eat large marine arthropods that are related to the smaller terrestrial arthropods we call insects. These marine arthropods—crabs, shrimp, and lobster—are delicious when eaten with melted butter. The arthropod family also includes crayfish, sowbugs and pillbugs, spiders, scorpions, millipedes, and centipedes.

Insects are an excellent source of protein. Our hunting and gathering ancestors certainly ate bugs in order to survive, and insects are still eaten by many people all over the world. The ancient Greeks and Romans dined quite well on insects. The Roman naturalist Pliny the Elder wrote that Roman aristocrats loved to eat beetle larvae that had been raised on flour and wine. The fourth-century B.C. Greek philosopher Aristotle wrote about techniques for harvesting the most delectable cicadas.

At least half the cultures in the world encourage insect-eating. In Ghana, winged termites are harvested during the spring rainy season and then eaten fried, roasted, or ground into flour and made into bread. In South Africa termites are eaten with cornmeal porridge. Chinese beekeepers regularly eat bee larvae from their hives. Japanese chefs sauté aquatic fly larvae with sugar and soy sauce. Roasted grubs are a delicacy in New Guinea and Australia. Cicadas, fire-roasted tarantulas, and ants are commonly added to traditional Latin American dishes. The most famous culinary insect of all, the agave "worm," is added to bottles of mezcal liquor in Mexico.

There are many nutritional and environmental benefits to entomophagy. Gene DeFoliart, a professor emeritus of entomology at the University of Wisconsin-Madison, stated: "In our preoccupation with cattle, we have denuded the planet of vegetation. Insects are much more efficient in converting biomass to protein," and added, "People are poisoning the planet by ridding it of insects, rather than eating insects and keeping artificial chemicals off plants that we eat." Insect ranching is much more efficient than cattle ranching: It takes one hundred pounds of feed to produce ten pounds of beef, while one hundred pounds of feed will produce forty-five pounds of crickets. Hamburger contains 18 percent protein and 18 percent fat. According to the table on the Iowa State website, whole crickets contain approximately 55 percent protein and 23 percent fat. Insect fats, like fish oils, are unsaturated.

Here are a couple of sites that feature recipes for cooking insects:

www.ent.iastate.edu/misc/insectsasfood (This Iowa State site features a table of the nutritional value of thirteen different insects, as well as recipes for Banana Worm Bread, Rootworm Beetle Dip, Chocolate Chirpie Chip Cookies, Crackers and Cheese Dip with Candied Crickets, Mealworm Fried Rice, Corn Borer Cornbread Muffins, and Chocolate-Covered Grasshoppers.)

www.eatbug.com (According to this website, there are 1,462 recorded species of edible insects. There are certainly many more edible species that haven't been sampled yet. This site also contains recipes as well as information on harvesting, raising, buying, and preparing edible insects.)

Two insect-eaters' cookbooks are *Man Eating Bugs: The Art and Science of Eating Insects* by Peter Menzel and Faith D'Alluisio (New York: Ten Speed Press, 1998)—an anthropological look at global entomophagy—and *The Eat a Bug Cookbook* by David George Gordon (New York: Ten Speed Press, 1998)—recipes by the author of *The Compleat Cockroach*.

I have inadvertently swallowed many innocent invertebrates that were living happily in grain products, fruits, or vegetables before I ingested them, or were flying around minding their own business until I came along and inhaled them. So far, the only type of insect I have eaten on purpose is roasted grasshopper, which is palatable but a bit bland; it cries out for barbecue sauce.

I was recently surprised to learn that grasshoppers, crickets, and locusts are the only invertebrates that are considered kosher: "Even these of them ye may eat; the locust after his kind, and the bald locust after his kind, and the beetle after his kind, and the grasshopper after his kind" (Leviticus, 11:22).

Sometimes after a plague of locusts has eaten every sprig of green in the landscape, the locusts are the only things left to eat.

## WASTED POTENTIAL

A few years ago I was in a fancy-food store in Chicago and was shocked and dismayed to see a basket full of astonishingly cheap garlic. (This garlic was so cheap, in fact, that I would not be able to sell my homegrown garlic at as low a price, even though I do all the work myself and have no overhead expenses: I produce my own fertilizer at home, dig my beds by hand, replant my own garlic cloves each year, and water the garlic with water dunked out of rain barrels.) Yet here was a whole basket full of little boxes of garlic, three heads for a quarter, that had been shipped all the way from China! The heads were certainly small, light, and rather dry, but they were garlic, and people were buying them.

In 2006, the average wholesale price of Chinese garlic in the United States was thirty-five cents per pound, but large volumes of Chinese garlic were also dumped on the market for as little as seven cents a pound. I grow approximately fifty pounds of garlic annually, which is just about enough to keep us happy for a year. If I decided to sell my entire fifty-pound garlic crop to our local co-op for Chinese prices, I could earn as much as $17.50 or as little as $3.50 for the lot. If I included the cost of driving the garlic into town, I would actually lose money by selling my garlic at the lowest price.

In 1994, at the instigation of the Fresh Garlic Producers Association, the United States imposed a 377 percent duty against fresh Chinese garlic. Before this duty was imposed, China had been selling its product for less than the cost of production, and this product dumping was harming the American garlic industry. Through the late 1990s, approximately one million pounds of Chinese garlic were imported into the United States each year. At the beginning of the twenty-first century, garlic imports began escalating; eighty-six million pounds of Chinese garlic were imported into the United States in 2004. American growers are again complaining that garlic importers are selling "dumped" garlic, critics claim that importers are taking advantage of a loophole in the legislation in order to circumvent the law. In 2006, for the very first time, garlic imported from China outsold garlic grown in California. Sales of Chinese garlic are booming, despite the fact that the Chinese garlic is an obviously inferior product that is lighter, drier, and less flavorful than domestically grown garlic.

Cheap Chinese garlic is being shipped all over the world, and all over the world, garlic farmers are going out of business because they are unable to compete with the ridiculously low price of Chinese garlic: California garlic growers cut their production from 160 million pounds of garlic in 2003 down to 95 million pounds in 2007.

Sue Kedgeley, MP, of New Zealand's Green Party, stated: "We have undercut the garlic industry via cheap garlic imports and that's just about wiped out—it's on its knees. . . . Only five garlic growers are left in New Zealand because cheap Chinese imports have severely undercut their market."

Thailand's garlic production dropped by more than 20 percent between 2004 and 2007.

And last but not least, in 2000, China temporarily suspended imports of South Korean cell phones and polyethylene in retaliation against Seoul's sharp increase in tariffs on garlic. In July 2002, Han Duck-Soo, South Korea's top presidential adviser on economic affairs, was forced to resign as Korean farmers protested against the influx of cheap Chinese garlic into their country. Mr. Han had been instrumental in lifting the restrictions on Chinese garlic two years previously.

The Chinese are not bestowing their cheap garlic upon the rest of the world out of the kindness of their hearts. The cheap garlic seems to be having its intended effect, and once the job is done, consumers may suddenly discover that the only garlic on the market is imported from China and that it is selling for grossly inflated prices.

## REQUIEM FOR A PROCESSING PLANT

At the beginning of the twenty-first century, De Francesco & Sons, Inc., of Firebaugh, California, was a successful, family-owned business, and one of the three major U.S. garlic processors. The company had been in business since 1968, running a 700,000-square-foot food dehydration plant, and 2,400 acres of San Joaquin Valley farmland on which they grew their own varieties of garlic, herbs, and vegetables to supply their processing plant. In 2006, De Francesco & Sons closed all its operations, driven out of business by cheap Chinese garlic.

The company will be sadly missed by its 187 former employees, as well as by the entire city of Firebaugh, California, estimated population 6,688. The closure was described as a devastating blow to the local economy.

It is terrible to lay waste to a community in this way.

The survivors hope that you will support your community by buying locally produced food and products.

## LOCAVORES

If a product has traveled halfway around the world before it reaches your local store, yet is drastically cheaper than its exact domestic equivalent, you can probably safely assume that something is not right at the other end. (But you have to compare apples to apples here. You cannot compare the price of organic produce to that of conventionally grown produce. You cannot compare greenhouse-grown produce to produce grown outdoors.) Cheapness is almost inevitably paid for with suffering; sometimes it is underpaid, pesticide-poisoned workers who suffer, sometimes individual consumers are harmed by dangerous products, often the environment is damaged, and sometimes an entire economy languishes.

It can be quite complicated to figure out which foods have the least impact on the environment. In general, any food that is grown locally, without large inputs of fossil fuel or petroleum-based fertilizers and pesticides, is the easiest on the environment. But the environmental equation can get quite complicated when it is dealing with out-of-season produce. For instance, shipping tomatoes or strawberries from a warm climate to a cold climate may use less fossil fuel than it would take to grow these same fruits in a heated greenhouse in a cold climate.

## DANGER IN THE HOME FIELDS

Most of the produce grown in the United States is harvested by migrant farmworkers, many of whom are in the country illegally. The workers' tenuous legal status makes them quite vulnerable to exploitation. Despite laws passed in 1988 requiring growers to provide drinking water and field toilets for their workers, many growers still do not do so.

According to the Centers for Disease Control and Prevention (CDC), the average American has a life expectancy of 77.2 years, but the average life expectancy of migrant farmworkers in the United States is 49 years. Most farmworkers have little or no access to medical care, and they have higher rates of diabetes, anemia, and hypertension, as well as tuberculosis, HIV/AIDS, parasitic infections, and other infectious diseases than the general population.

Harvesting produce is backbreaking, heartbreaking, and often toxic work. I have watched farmworkers in action, and I am fairly certain that even though I am well accustomed to hard, outdoor labor, I would not last even a single day harvesting Brussels sprouts or artichokes.

A lot of cheap lettuce is harvested by workers who have no access to drinking water or to toilet or hand-washing facilities. Since those workers have a very high incidence of dangerous communicable diseases and parasitic infections, and occasionally drop in the fields from heat exhaustion and pesticide poisoning, how safe can that lettuce be? The answer is:

not very. Many researchers have found that *E. coli* O157:H7 and *Salmonella typhimurium* bacteria can live in the inner tissues of lettuce leaves and other leafy greens, as well as in soft fruits such as tomatoes and melons. The researchers also discovered that the plants' leaves absorb the bacteria directly from their surfaces, or the root system can efficiently transport the bacteria to the rest of the plant. Once inside, the bacteria cannot be washed off the produce. We're all in this together, folks! Misery spreads.

Moral: You get what you pay for, but if you don't pay much, what you get might not be what you want.

### ORGANIZATIONS

The Fair Trade movement works to improve the lives of workers worldwide by securing workers' rights and increasing their share of profits. The Fair Trade label on products is a signal that Fair Trade standards were adhered to and the people who worked to produce that product were not exploited. For more information, go to:

Fairtrade Labeling Organizations International (FLO): www.fairtrade.net. The FLO sets Fair Trade standards, inspects producers, and ensures compliance to Fair Trade standards. Producers that are in compliance can affix the Fair Trade Certification mark to their products.

Fair Trade Federation: www.fairtradefederation.org. Listings of retailers, wholesalers, distributors, and producers who are committed to selling items that are produced following the Fair Trade guidelines.

United Farm Workers Union: www.ufw.org. The UFW has fought long and hard to improve working conditions, gain basic human rights, and reduce pesticide exposure for migrant farmworkers in the United States. Every time a battle is won, our food supply gets a little bit safer.

And now for something completely obvious: Businesses are in business to make a profit. A business that does not make a profit will eventually go out of business—thus has it ever been. Every single person who handles a product between the time it is produced until it reaches its final purchaser wants to make a profit from the transaction. The farther a product travels, the greater the number of people who have earned money by handling it. Processed and ready-to-eat foods are the products of many people's labor, and all of the people who have worked with that food want to be paid. According to a report released in 2006 by the Department of Agriculture, labor accounts for 38.5 percent of all food costs in the United States, packaging adds another 8 percent to overall food costs, and advertising adds another 8 percent.

In the first quarter of 2008, farmers received $5.50 per bushel of corn, while an 18-ounce box of corn flakes cost approximately $3.30 and contained approximately 7.9 cents' worth of corn, and there was 16 cents' worth of wheat in a 20-ounce loaf of bread that retailed for $1.78.

If you want to spend the minimum amount possible on healthy food, learn to cook, buy as much of your food in bulk as possible, bring your own containers, and whenever possible, buy directly from the farmer. It is pure illusion that junk food and fast food are cheap. Someone has to pay for the advertising, labor, and packaging that went into that food, and we are that someone. When every red cent counts, why pay for packaging that is used once, then thrown away?

If you are one of the fortunate few who can buy whatever you want, whenever you want to, please try to buy locally grown, organically grown food as much as possible because it is vital that we keep our local food producers and small farmers in business. Otherwise, we will all eventually be at the mercy of Big Agribusinesses.

Save a small farmer, save the world.

## SOUL FOOD

Spend your time and money acquiring unique experiences rather than mass-produced stuff. Sing, dance, write, create art. Attend live performances. Buy art directly from the artist. Buy books while their authors are still alive.

Save an artist, save our culture.

## CHAPTER THREE

# The Barbarian's Kitchen

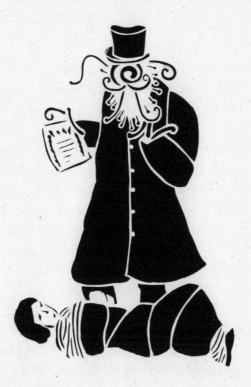

This chapter will not tell you how to have the most blindingly shiny kitchen on your block. This book is about living bravely and healthily, and keeping oneself ready to fight the good fight against those who would take advantage of us and control us. As Sun Tzu said in *The Art of War*: "Do not swallow bait offered by the enemy." Easy, envy-inducing prettiness and cleanliness is the bait that Big Business is dangling in front of us, but like a lot of bait, it is made of scented plastic and will not nourish us.

This chapter deals with running a shipshape kitchen so you can avoid producing crops of homegrown food poisoning. But all that gleams isn't necessarily health-inducing, and dull and worn isn't necessarily dangerous. Clean is not in the eye of the beholder, unless that beholder happens to be looking through a microscope.

## CHOOSING YOUR POISON

The Centers for Disease Control and Prevention (CDC) informs us that millions of Americans are afflicted by food poisoning every year. The USDA is so concerned about food safety that in the spring of 2007 it hosted a Food Safety camp for children. The young campers enjoyed fun activities such as a glow-in-the-dark hand-washing demonstration, and studied food-poisoning bacteria through a high-powered microscope. They also learned about the importance of keeping hot foods hot and cold foods cold, how to pack and store bag lunches, and were drilled in the key messages associated with the USDA's Be Food Safe Campaign: Clean, Separate, Cook, and Chill.

Perhaps the U.S. Food and Drug Administration (FDA), which is responsible for regulating about 80 percent of the food sold in the United States, as well as all drugs, human vaccines, and medical devices, should hire some of these newly trained food safety experts to help beef up its ranks.

According to a report released in December 2007, the FDA is woefully underfunded and understaffed. The report, titled "FDA Science and Mission at Risk: Report of the Subcommittee on Science and Technology," states baldly that "American lives are at risk." The subcommittee found that the FDA is so pathetically understaffed, underequipped, and underfunded that safety inspectors write their reports out by hand rather than on computers, food-processing plants are inspected once every ten years (at best), only two employees work full time on pet-food safety, and the only copies of many critically important information are paper documents that are piled in locked warehouses.

The report states: "We found that FDA's resource shortfalls have resulted in a plethora of inadequacies that threaten our society—including, but not limited to, inadequate inspections of manufacturers, a dearth of scientists who understand emerging new technologies, inability to speed the development of new therapies, an import system that is badly broken, a food supply that grows riskier each year, and an information infrastructure that was identified as a source of risk in every Center and program reviewed by the Subcommittee. . . . The report suggests the agency may need as much as twice its current level of funding to equip it properly to fulfill its mission."

I wonder if the Food Safety campers were taught what to do with frozen Chinese fish that were raised in contaminated water and fed banned antibiotics? Or what to do with a puffed rice and corn snack that is coated with vegetable-flavored salmonella? Or how to deal with a pet that has been sickened by melamine-contaminated pet food?

## HAND WASHING

Since the FDA seems to have misplaced its mission, it's more important than ever that we know how to reduce our risk of food poisoning.

The three tines of food safety are: to acquire clean, healthful food; to avoid contaminating it after one has acquired it; and to prepare and store it properly so it stays clean and healthful. The first step in that direction is to wash one's hands before preparing food.

A tiny army, composed of millions of bacteria, fungi, and viruses, lives on your hands (and mine, and everyone else's). Most of these microbes are necessary and permanent residents that help protect the skin from dangerous pathogens.

Obviously, a product that could remove hitchhiking pathogens while leaving our resident microbes intact would be a great boon to health. Fortunately for all of us, this fabulous product has already been invented. It's called soap.

## THE NEW WAVE OF HAND WASHING

Many newfangled products advertised as more effective than plain old soap and water have flooded the market. Some of them have become quite popular.

In the United States, up to 75 percent of all liquid soaps and 30 percent of bar soaps now contain antimicrobials, which would not be such a bad thing if there were any evidence at all that antimicrobial soaps are actually safe and more effective. But there is none. Study after study has shown that plain soap and water are just as effective at killing and removing bacteria from the skin as antimicrobial soaps. Even that would not be so bad if there was not so much evidence that antimicrobials are damaging the environment and endangering our health.

A 2002 study conducted by the U.S. Geological Survey found that triclosan and phthalates from antimicrobial soaps are polluting waterways across the United States. Some phthalates are known endocrine disrupters that may cause severe reproductive problems and birth defects in both wildlife and humans. The solution to this problem is not to buy more bottled water, it is to choose and use products that are free of these toxins. Municipal water systems are far more carefully regulated and inspected than are water-bottling plants.

Triclosan is the most common antimicrobial found in consumer products such as dish liquids, soap, lotion, shampoo, toothpaste, and cosmetics; it is highly toxic to fish and crustaceans as well as to the algae and bacteria that are crucial to the survival of aquatic ecosystems. When it is exposed to sunlight, triclosan breaks down and is converted to a dioxin. Dioxins are endocrine disrupters that are persistent in the environment. And when triclosan is exposed to hot, chlorinated water, it produces chloroform gas, which may make the steam emanating from a sinkful of hot dishwater a little too relaxing to be healthy.

## BE KIND TO YOUR FINE MICROBIAL FRIENDS

Exposure to antimicrobial products may kill the friendly bacteria that help us digest and absorb our food. Our health and well-being depend on the vitamins (K, $B_{12}$, thiamine, and riboflavin) that our beneficial, symbiotic bacteria synthesize in our guts. Antimicrobials may also kill, damage, or discourage the resident bacteria that protect our skin by outcompeting dangerous microbes. Almost inevitably, when we target chemicals at dangerous organisms, the offensive organisms—whether animal, vegetable, or microbe—quickly adapt and evolve resistance to the poison, while the resident beneficials quietly succumb.

Laboratory tests have shown that dangerous microbes are developing resistance to antimicrobials such as triclosan, and there is some concern that the use of antimicrobials is also contributing to the evolution of antibiotic-resistant bacteria such as penicillin-resistant *Streptococcus pneumoniae*, vancomycin-resistant enterococci, multiresistant salmonella, methicillin-resistant *Staphylococcus aureus*, and multiresistant *Mycobacterium tuberculosis*. These microbes cause pneumonia, food poisoning, skin lesions, and tuberculosis. Antibiotic-resistant bacteria tend to be even more virulent and dangerous than the original versions—our fear of microbes, and our consequent overuse, misuse, and abuse of antibiotics and antimicrobials are creating microbial monsters. In 2002, the American Medical Association released a report that stated: "it is prudent to avoid the use of antimicrobial agents in consumer products."

Unfortunately, the liquid soaps we encounter in public bathrooms are very likely to contain antimicrobials. So how does one avoid using antimicrobial liquid soaps in public bathrooms? Sylvia Garcia-Houchins, manager of infection control at the University of Chicago Medical Center, suggests just rubbing your hands together under warm running water. The scrubbing action does the job. Drying your hands thoroughly and vigorously afterward on a paper towel will wipe out the rest of the transient bacteria.

## PICKLED HANDS: SOUSED NOROVIRUSES

Alcohol-based hand-washing gels have been used in hospitals for quite a few years, and it was assumed that these gels were as good as, if not better than, using plain old soap and water for removing dangerous bacteria and viruses from the hands of medical workers. But in 2006, Christine Moe of Emory University in Atlanta, Georgia, tested the efficacy of alcohol-based hand gels against noroviruses—viruses that cause acute gastrointestinal illness (perhaps most notoriously on cruise ships). Moe and her colleagues spread a carefully measured quantity of a norovirus on the fingers of volunteers, and then cleaned three of each volunteer's fingers with either antibacterial soap, plain water, or an alcohol-based hand sanitizer. The volunteers' remaining fingers were left unwashed for comparison.

The researchers were surprised to find that plain water killed 96 percent of the Norwalk virus, antibacterial soap killed 88 percent of the virus, and the alcohol-based hand gels killed about half of the virus. Moe said that alcohol-based gels "are better than nothing, but in areas where soap and water are available, people should use them first."

## CROCKED CLOSTRIDIUM

Alcohol-based hand cleaners are nearly useless against some dangerous bacteria. A 2007 study conducted by Dr. Michael Oughton, of McGill University in Canada, found that washing with an alcohol-based hand cleaner eliminated almost no *Clostridium difficile* bacteria. *C. difficile* can cause illnesses ranging from diarrhea to life-threatening inflammation of the colon in people who are taking antacids, antibiotics, or other antimicrobial drugs that upset the normal flora in the intestine. *C. difficile* is responsible for tens of thousands of cases of diarrhea and at least five thousand deaths every year in the United States. Virulent antibiotic-resistant strains of *C. difficile* are rapidly evolving. These superbugs can produce potent toxins that attack the lining of the intestines, killing cells and rotting the interior. *C. difficile* is commonly transported from victim to victim on unwashed hands.

Dr. Oughton's team contaminated volunteers' hands with *C. difficile*, then cleaned their hands using five different hand-washing protocols: plain soap and warm or cold water; antiseptic soap with warm water; an alcohol-based solution; and a disinfectant towel. Said Oughton: "The results were striking: the protocols that involved washing with water eliminated more than 98 per cent of the bacteria, while washing with an alcohol-based solution eliminated almost none."

If you want to stay healthy, wash your hands with plain soap and water. You only want to remove the transient microbes from your skin, not the friendly, permanent residents.

## TRIM YOUR CLAWS

A study conducted by the Oklahoma State Health Department, the Centers for Disease Control and Prevention, and Children's Hospital of Oklahoma found that bacteria lurking under the long fingernails of two nurses may have contributed to the deaths of sixteen frail premature babies at Children's Hospital of Oklahoma in 1997 and 1998.

The CDC studied the records of all the babies who were admitted to the Neonatal Intensive Care Unit in 1997 and the first part of 1998. Of the 439 newborns who were admitted during that period, 46 acquired a *Pseudomonas aeruginosa* infection and 16 died. The babies who were infected were cared for by two nurses who had long or artificial fingernails. Even chipped fingernail polish harbors significant quantities of bacteria.

The hospital now requires all nurses to wear their fingernails short and natural.

## BARBARIAN HARDWARE

Not only have advertisers convinced us that we should live in fear of the dangerous microbes on our hands, skin, and nails, but now they've gone even further, and we must commence worrying about the bacterial dangers lurking on our kitchen surfaces—from countertops to cutting boards to drawer handles. The truth is that there have always been microbes on our planet, and there always will be. Few microbes are capable of surviving, much less multiplying, on hard, dry surfaces, and even fewer are capable of jumping out at you from these surfaces.

## GETTING A HANDLE ON IT

Occasionally microbes that cling to objects can, and do, migrate to uninfected people and make them ill—especially in hospitals. Because of the use, overuse, and abuse of antibiotics and antimicrobials, hospitals have become breeding grounds for dangerous supermicrobes that are resistant to treatment.

Several years ago an elderly friend of mine was hospitalized, and during my many visits to her, I was horrified to discover that despite the fact that public health experts were inveighing against antimicrobial soaps and lotions because of the danger of producing "superbugs," all the bathrooms in the hospital were supplied with antimicrobial soap.

Because my friend developed a life-threatening infection while in the hospital, and her stay was prolonged by a month, I had plenty of time to ponder the situation. I did a bit of research, and discovered that copper, bronze, and brass all have antimicrobial properties. A study conducted in 2000, at the Centre for Applied Microbiology & Research (CAMR) in the U.K., found that the dangerous *E. coli* O157 strain survived for much shorter periods of time on copper and brass surfaces than it did on stainless steel. The research team found that at room temperature, *E. coli* O157 survived for thirty-four days on a stainless-steel surface. The bacteria lived for four days on brass, and just four hours on copper. When refrigerated, the bacteria survived longer than thirty-four days on stainless steel, twelve days on brass, and fourteen hours on copper.

> *E. coli* O157 is a highly infectious pathogen that can cause diarrhea, nausea, colitis, kidney disease, and death. It infects tens of thousands of people worldwide every year. The bacteria can be found in meat, water, dairy products, and raw fruit and vegetable juices. Infection can also result from contact with an *E. coli*–infected person.

A 2005 study conducted at the University of Southampton, U.K., showed that methicillin-resistant *Staphylococcus aureus* (MRSA) stayed alive for up to seventy-two hours on stainless steel, though it succumbed after only an hour and a half on a copper surface. Alloys containing various amounts of copper killed the antibiotic-resistant bacteria at rates directly proportional to the amount of copper they contained—the more copper, the faster the kill. Tests conducted with bacterial concentrations that more closely mimicked those found in real life showed that copper surfaces completely eliminated all live MRSA and *E. coli* bacteria in twenty minutes. Dr. Bill Keevil, the head of the university's environmental health care unit, said: "Our results strongly indicate that use of the copper metals in such applications as door knobs, push plates, fittings, fixtures and work surfaces would considerably mitigate MRSA in hospitals and reduce the risk of cross-contamination between staff and patients in critical care areas." Another study, which was also conducted at the University of Southhamptom showed that copper, brass, and bronze surfaces also kill *Clostridium difficile* bacteria and its spores.

I was more germphobic during that month of hospital visits than I have ever been before or since. Surrounded by multitudes of sick people, and facing the malevolent gleam of stainless-steel door handles, elevator buttons, faucet handles, stair railings, and bed rails, I longed for the warm, friendly glow of brass, bronze, or copper. I used my sleeve to open and close doors and to push elevator buttons; I scalded my hands with hot water rather than use the hospital's antimicrobial liquid soaps. After each visit, I longed to rid myself of the hospital miasma by rolling in the dirt like a dog; I usually contented myself with plunging my arms up to the elbow in my worm composting bins, cleaning out the chicken coop, or eating carrots from our garden without washing them first.

The use of clean-looking, easily washed stainless steel, plastic, and aluminum in hospitals is a triumph of style over substance. For many years, it was assumed that gleaming stainless steel was the most hygienic surface for medical facilities, because it looked so clean compared to the more old-fashioned, tarnished appearance of brass railings, which eventually acquire a patina that many people interpret as "dirty." It all depends on your definition of "clean." If clean means shining, unstained, and untarnished, then yes, stainless steel is clean. On the other hand, if clean means not tending to induce illness, then even the most tarnished and dull brass, bronze, or copper handle is cleaner than the shiniest stainless-steel handle.

If you are concerned about microbes in your kitchen or bathroom, install brass, bronze, or copper handles!

## GNARLY WOOD

According to research conducted in 1992 by Philip H. Kass at the University of California–Davis, people who use bright, shiny glass or plastic cutting boards are twice as likely to get salmonella poisoning as people who use wooden cutting boards. Research conducted by Dean O. Cliver and Nese O. Ak showed why: Wood fibers absorb and kill bacteria within three minutes. The knife scars in plastic and glass cutting boards make comfortable little breeding ponds for bacteria, and neither cycling through the dishwasher nor being heated in the microwave will dislodge bacteria from their plastic or glass ponds.

But what, one may ask, about the plastic Microban cutting boards that are permanently impregnated with the antimicrobial triclosan? Wouldn't they prevent bacterial growth? Research published in 2001 by Herbert P. Schweizer, a microbiologist at Colorado State University in Fort Collins, showed that the mutations that have allowed bacteria such as *Mycobacterium tuberculosis* and *Pseudomonas aeruginosa* (which frequently infect hospital patients) to develop resistance to triclosan, have also made these bacteria resistant to many antibiotics.

What could possibly be more fulfilling and exciting than breeding your very own strain of food poisoning "superbugs" in and on your own cutting board? If you are in a rush, perhaps you could speed up the evolutionary process by installing a Microban sink and countertops and using Microban-laced kitchen sponges!

## WHAT IS CLEAN?

I am an enthusiastic housework shirker; if there is a safe way to avoid or speed up any specific household task, I want to know about it. So when I read about the research done by Professors Chuck Gerba and Carlos Enriques of the University of Arizona at Tucson, I was entranced. Gerba and Enriques analyzed samples from one thousand private kitchens in five American cities and discovered that the average kitchen sink is more likely to be harboring dangerous bacteria than is the average toilet bowl, the average kitchen floor is cleaner than the average kitchen counter, and the cleaner-looking the kitchen, the more likely it was to have dangerous bacteria all over it.

Why, one may well ask, are the cleanest-looking kitchens the most heavily contaminated? The explanation for these seemingly inexplicable results is that the cleanest-looking kitchens are usually those that are frequently swabbed down with that most dangerous of all household implements: the kitchen sponge. Kitchen sponges are porous objects that take a full two weeks to completely dry out, and during those moist two weeks, bacteria multiply continuously. All that gleams is not necessarily clean. Said Gerba, "Bachelors don't clean often, so they don't contaminate things with a dirty dishrag."

## STOP SPONGING

As soon as I read about the dangers of kitchen sponges, I threw ours away and went out and bought several dozen dishcloths. I put a small laundry basket near the kitchen, and we now wash a load of kitchen linens, which includes our cloth napkins, tablecloths, and dishcloths, about once a week in hot water. This routine works very well, because most of our other laundry is washed in either cool or warm water, which is not as effective at removing grease.

The dishcloths get us through a whole week of dishwashing and countertop swabbing without my ever having to use an already damp, bacteria-laden dishcloth to wipe down a counter or wash a dish. I just use a clean, dry cloth every time.

If you have limited access to a washer and dryer, find somewhere that you can hang your dishcloths up to dry. Each time you wash your dishes, rinse your dishcloth out very thoroughly, wring it out as well as you can, then hang it up to dry. Use a dry dishcloth each time you wash the dishes or wipe the counter, and do not reuse a dishcloth until it is completely dry. This will cut down on your volume of kitchen laundry.

## WIPING UP

Any cleaning job that doesn't actually require toilet paper is probably better accomplished with a reusable or reused cloth. Old worn-out rags can be used to tackle truly filthy jobs—for instance, those involving housepaint, engine grease, or unhousebroken puppies—and can then be disposed of. Less drastically filthy cleaning jobs can be accomplished efficiently, cleanly, and cheaply with washable, reusable towels or rags.

Cleaning jobs that are done privately do not require pretty cleaning rags. Any clean, absorbent cloth can be used to clean mirrors and windows, dust furniture and knickknacks, and wash floors and walls. We are still polishing things and wiping up messes with the cloth diapers our children wore twenty years ago. Old T-shirts, worn-out sheets, and holey socks make lovely absorbent and lint-free reusable, disposable, or compostable rags. Even old blue jeans can be used when a really tough, slightly abrasive rag is called for.

Though I am a huge fan of ancient, holey rags, even I balk at using old diapers or pieces of old T-shirts as table napkins, so every couple of years we buy pretty new dishcloths or washcloths to be used as everyday napkins, and when these everyday napkins get ragged, we demote them to dish duty. We also own a few sets of "company" napkins that we use when we have guests.

## CLASSICAL NAPKINS

The ancient Greeks wiped their hands on scraps of bread while they dined, and after the meal they washed their hands with water. The ancient Romans used cloth napkins, but by the early Middle Ages, Europeans had abandoned table napkins and tended to wipe on anything they could reach, including the backs of their hands, their clothes, or a piece of bread.

Later in the Middle Ages, table manners improved, and each table was laid with a large cloth that was used as a communal napkin. By the sixteenth century, the individual cloth napkin had been reintroduced.

In 1907, a shipment of extrathick paper was delivered to the Scott Paper Company. The paper was too thick to be made into toilet paper, but rather than send the entire shipment back, the head of the company invented the paper towel. The paper napkin made its debut a few decades later.

I think the road to hell is being paved with disposables (so is a large swath of the southern Pacific Ocean, which is now known as the Great Pacific Garbage Patch, or trash vortex, a stew of floating plastic garbage that is twice the size of the continental United States). However, some occasions simply cry out for tableware and napkins that do not need to be washed afterward. Biodegradable plates, cups, and flatware made from unbleached paper and/or bioplastics derived from plants are better alternatives than noncompostable plastic tableware. Note: These products must be either sent to a municipal compost facility or be put in a backyard compost pile in order to decompose. If they are interred in a landfill, they will last forever.

Here are some sources for biodegradable table settings. For the beautiful and unusual:

Eatitworld (www.eatitworld.com) is a design company that produces beautiful and amusing cutting-edge products from highly unusual materials. Their Botanika Leafware is made from tropical leaves that are woven together with natural fibers and formed into plates, bowls, place mats, and table covers.

For the utilitarian:

Sinless Buying (www.sinlessbuying.com) sells paper plates, trays, cups, bowls, and boxes made from sugarcane bagasse (the fibers that are left after the sugarcane juice is extracted) and starch-based flatware.

Worldcentric (www.worldcentric.org) sells biodegradable plates, trays, bowls, cups, and food containers made of bagasse, as well as cups and flatware made of bioplastics.

## THE NEW-AGE CLEAN PLATE CLUB

Rather than setting his banquet table with expensive compostables, the thrifty Green Barbarian may opt to eat his table setting in the medieval manner.

The medieval diner ate his meal from a trencher, a plate that was cut from a specially baked loaf of bread that was allowed to go stale before it was put into service. After the meal, the used trenchers, which were dotted with bits of food and soaked with sauces and gravies, were customarily thrown to the household dogs or presented to the poor. The big eaters who finished their meal and then ate the plate were called trenchermen.

## BREAD BOWLS

Trenchermen must have been extremely hungry in order to want to eat their stale, coarse trenchers. However, the trencher's modern relative, the bread bowl, is quite tasty. Chili, thick soups, and stews are all delicious when served in bread bowls, and most people happily finish off their bowls after ingesting their contents.

The modern bread bowl is usually a small, round loaf of crusty, resilient French, Italian, or sourdough bread that has had its top sliced off and its inside hollowed out.

Brush the interior of the hollow bread bowl with olive oil or butter, then bake it at 400 degrees for five minutes, or until golden, to make the bread bowl more moisture-resistant.

The bread torn out of the inside of the bread bowl can be cut into cubes and used for croutons, poultry stuffing, or bread pudding. Or you can just butter and eat it.

## MODERN BREAD NAPKINS

Many of my friends do not mind being used as human guinea pigs. Recently, in order to test the properties of various types of bread, I sent out the following invitation:

*Hello Friends!*

*We are having a party this Sunday, July 6th, from three until whenever. I want to use as many friends as possible to help me test out the concept of "bread napkins" for my book. Toward that end we are throwing a "messy party," and will be serving really messy food along with breadlike items that are very springy (French bread would be a good example) that we can use to wipe the grease, barbecue sauce, and salad dressing off our faces and hands.*

*If you want to bring something, I humbly request that you bring either a food that is extremely messy, OR a springy bread of some kind (along with the recipe or the information about where to get it).*

*Casual clothing, and/or bibs and/or aprons are suggested! We have a badminton net, horseshoes, Frisbees, and a very frisky puppy.*

*Hope to see you there!*
*Ellen and Walt*

The party was a roaring success. The guests arrived in play clothes, some sporting jaunty aprons, and carrying armloads of delicious food. We gorged on gooey barbecued ribs, saucy chicken, pulled chicken rolled in tortillas, corn on the cob, fry bread, rye bread, wheat bread, egg bread, English muffins, pasta salad, green salad, strawberries and whipping cream, gingerbread, and blueberries in Jell-O, and ate in the delicate medieval manner: with our hands.

The unrivaled champion in the bread napkin contest was the homely tortilla, followed closely by the resilient *New York Times* No Knead Bread. The English muffin had the correct texture but had an unfortunate tendency to leave a dusting of flour on the user's face and hands (the next batch of English muffins will be dusted with cornmeal, not with flour). The egg bread was far too crumbly to function as a napkin at all.

The fry bread was the unchallenged winner in the bread plate division, and worked quite well when placed on a bamboo paper-plate holder.

One guest brought birchbark scraps—she thought the suedelike inner surface of the birchbark might come in handy.

At the end of the meal, another guest emptied her water glass over her hands, then dried them on a piece of birchbark. The dampened birchbark was passed along, and worked quite well as a grease-absorbing napkin.

If you decide to use bread napkins, there are several options for disposing of bread that has been wiped on.

1. You can eat it. If you think this is unsanitary, you should have washed your hands before you ate.
2. You can follow medieval custom and throw it to the dogs. (Used bread was also thrown to the starving peasants, but we maintain optimism that our economy is not going to sink that low.)
3. You can feed it to ducks, chickens, swans, or even pigeons.
4. You can put it in a freezer bag and save it to thicken soups or stews. If this strikes you as disgusting, please reread item #1.
5. You can compost it.

## WIPING TIPS

It is probably not surprising that the tortillas won the napkin contest. All over the world there are variations on the multipurpose flatbread theme, and using flatbreads as napkins is a common practice. A few examples include Ethiopian injera, a large, crepelike flatbread that is used as a table covering, a plate, a utensil to scoop up food, and a napkin; Indian flatbreads, such as chapati, phulka, roti, and parantha, used to scoop up or manipulate food; pita bread, used as a food wrap and eating utensil in Middle Eastern and Mediterranean countries; and in the New World, the ubiquitous tortilla, used for almost everything connected with food.

### TORTILLA MEMORIES, BY SUSIE NEWMAN

"While living and working in Mexico in the 1980s, my husband and I noticed how versatile the tortilla was. Besides the usual practice of putting meat and other fixings inside a tortilla, we also saw the humble tortilla used as a hotpad to protect the hands while picking up a hot pot; as a trivet to protect the table from a hot pot; rolled up and used as a spoon to eat soup or whatever dish was being served; and at the end of the meal a fresh tortilla was grabbed and used as a napkin to wipe the hands and mouth."

## A COUPLE OF BREAD NAPKIN RECIPES

This No Knead Bread recipe was featured in the *New York Times* on November 8, 2006. It quickly became a sensation and caused a temporary yeast shortage in New York City. The recipe in the *Times* was adapted from a recipe developed by Jim Lahey of the Sullivan Street Bakery. This recipe has been adapted from the recipe in the *Times*.

### LAZY BREAD FOR NAPKINS

Very moist, sticky bread doughs expand easily as carbon dioxide is released from rapidly growing yeast. If a dough is wet enough, kneading is not necessary in order to develop the gluten that will help the bread maintain its loft. During a long, slow rise in a very wet dough, the gluten molecules line up on their own and bind themselves together to produce a strong, elastic network that traps the carbon dioxide bubbles and prevents the bread from collapsing. Lower-moisture doughs must be kneaded in order to align the gluten molecules, which cannot travel easily through stiffer, drier dough.

This recipe produces a very wet dough that time and the oven metamorphose into a delicious, resilient bread that is just perfect for bread napkin duty.

Ingredients

*3-plus cups all-purpose or bread flour*
*$1/4$ teaspoon yeast*
*$1^1/4$ teaspoons salt*
*Wheat flour, cornmeal, or wheat bran for dusting the dough (use cornmeal*
*if you will be using the bread as a napkin)*

Equipment

*Mixing bowl*
*Measuring cups and spoons*

*Wooden spoon*
*Clean, smooth cotton kitchen towel (not terry cloth)*
*Heavy 6- or 8-quart covered pot*

Mix 3 cups of flour, the yeast, and the salt in a large bowl. Add 1⅝ cups of water, and stir until blended. The dough will be very sticky. Cover the bowl with plastic wrap and let it rest at warm room temperature (70 degrees) for at least 12 hours, though 18 hours is better.

The dough is ready to work when its surface is dotted with bubbles. Put the dough on a lightly floured work surface. Sprinkle the dough with a little more flour and fold it over a couple of times. Cover the folded dough loosely with plastic wrap and let it rest for about 15 minutes.

Sprinkle just enough flour on the dough to keep it from sticking to your work surface and your fingers, and gently and quickly shape the dough into a ball. Coat a smooth, napless cotton towel with a generous layer of flour, wheat bran, or cornmeal, then put the seam side of the dough down on the towel. Dust the dough with more flour, bran, or cornmeal, then fold the towel over the dough and allow the dough to rest for two hours. The dough is ready when it has more than doubled in size and stays dented when you poke it.

At least half an hour before the dough will be ready, put a 6- to 8-quart heavy covered pot (cast iron, enamel, or ceramic) in the oven, and preheat the oven to 450 degrees. When the dough is ready, carefully remove the pot from the oven and put it on top of the stove.

Slide your hand under the towel and flop the dough seam side up into the pot. Shake the pot a couple of times in order to center the dough. Though the dough may look rather disheveled at this stage, do not worry—it will rise in the oven and will shape up nicely.

Cover the pot with the lid, put it in the oven, and bake it covered for 30 minutes, then remove the lid and bake the bread uncovered for another 15 to 30 minutes, until the loaf is nicely browned. Cool the bread on a rack.

Note: It can be difficult to find a warm place for bread to rise during the summer when one is trying to keep one's home cool, so here are a few suggestions: inside a car parked in the sun on a warm day; on top of the refrigerator; behind the computer; and if you own a cat, watch where it lounges, because that spot is usually the warmest place in the house.

## CIABATTA RECIPE

This flattish Italian bread is springy and absorbent.

> *5 cups flour*
> *2 cups water*
> *1 or 2 packages yeast*
> *1 tablespoon sugar*
> *1 teaspoon salt*
> *1 tablespoon olive oil*

Combine all the ingredients except the olive oil. Place the dough in a bowl that has been greased with olive oil, cover, and let the dough rise until doubled in size.

Shape the dough into 3 flat rounds. Put the rounds on a pizza stone or a greased cookie sheet.

Bake at 350 degrees for 15 minutes.

## DISHWASHERS

Like death and taxes, dirty dishes are inevitable. Interestingly, dishwashing is one of the few human activities that is easier on the environment if done by machine.

Energy-efficient automatic dishwashers are so good at their job that they use far less water, energy, and dish detergent than even the most conscientious person would use while washing the same amount of dishes by hand. So if you have a dishwasher, use it! (If you have been forgoing the dishwasher and spending hours every day doing the dishes by hand as a form of penance, try to find another, more ecological way to atone for your sins.) Here are some ways to further increase the efficiency of your dishwasher.

The most efficient dishwashers have built-in water heaters. Let your dishwasher heat its own water to scalding temperatures and keep your house water heater set at a safer, energy-conserving 120 degrees F.

Run your dishwasher only when it is full. Consult the manufacturer's manual for advice on the best way to load the dishwasher so that you don't block the spray from hitting some of your dishes. If you have lost your manual, you may be able to download it from the manufacturer's website. General rules for loading a dishwasher include:

1. Scrape the large chunks of food off the dishes. Remove all hardened food as well as bits of cheese and egg, which the heat may melt onto the plate. Do not "prewash" the dishes before loading them into the dishwasher. Most modern dish detergents contain enzymes that break down food residues. If the enzymes don't have anything to do, they remain hard and abrasive and will effectively sandblast your dishes and glassware, removing decorative glazes and gilding, and making glassware permanently cloudy.

2. Use the minimum recommended amount of dish detergent. Too much detergent will leave a residue on the dishes.

3. Do not put wooden-handled knives in the dishwasher. The handles will eventually be ruined and the knives will fall apart. Dishwashers are not good for sharp knives in general. Wash them by hand.

4. Load knives and forks into the utensil basket with the sharp end down.

5. Choose "air drying" rather than the "heated drying" cycle. When the wash cycle is over, open the dishwasher and allow the dishes to air-dry before you put them away.

## KITCHEN GERM KILLERS

Recommended materials:

Plain, unscented dish liquid, which contains only ingredients that you can both pronounce and understand and is free of phosphates, chlorine, fragrance, and antimicrobials. (Does anyone really need dishes that smell like perfume?)

Distilled white vinegar in a spray bottle.

A bottle of hydrogen peroxide. (Drugstore strength, please! Chemical lab–strength hydrogen peroxide is a powerful oxidizer that can cause organic materials to spontaneously combust.)

Screw a spray nozzle on top of the bottle of hydrogen peroxide. Most spray nozzles for bottles will fit on a hydrogen peroxide bottle.

Do not decant the hydrogen peroxide into a light-colored, translucent, or transparent spray bottle. A hydrogen peroxide molecule is essentially a water molecule with an extra, very tenuously connected oxygen atom. This extra oxygen atom is easily dislodged from the rest of the molecule, which is what gives hydrogen peroxide its microbe-killing punch. The loose atom oxidizes and kills any microbes it encounters. But this means that if you expose hydrogen peroxide to light, leave the bottle uncapped, or shake the bottle, you will end up with a bottle of plain old water.

Question: If using antimicrobial dish liquid is a bad idea, and disinfecting the sink with chlorine is bad for the environment, how does one go about discouraging bacteria in the kitchen sink after one has rinsed off fresh produce or a raw chicken?

Answer: Squirt plain, unscented dish liquid on a clean dishcloth and use it to swab down the sink and faucet handles. Then spray the sink and faucet handles with white distilled vinegar and hydrogen peroxide. The order in which you spray does not matter. Do not mix vinegar and peroxide together in a bottle, or you will end up with watery vinegar.

The vinegar and peroxide sprays can be used to decontaminate produce, meat, and poultry. The combination can also be used to decontaminate countertops, as well as handles and doorknobs that you may have slopped with raw chicken juices during your food-rinsing frenzy.

## POISONED BY GREED

Culturing the bacteria that cause food poisoning is easier than falling off a log, because in order to culture food poisoning bacteria, you literally have to do nothing. Avoiding food poisoning is relatively easy if you follow all the rules taught to the Food Scouts. Unfortunately, avoiding being poisoned by greed may be a lot more difficult. In the past few years we have learned, sometimes the hard way, that cheap imports sometimes contain toxic ingredients. We have also learned that food that has been produced in a polluted area or in a contaminated facility may be cheap, but it will not be healthy. As they say, you get what you pay for.

Note: A more encyclopedic treatment of kitchen cleaning, including aesthetic cleaning, can be found in my previous book, *Organic Housekeeping*, which is known as *Green Housekeeping* in its paperback incarnation.

## KEEP YOUR POWDER DRY

The keys to kitchen hygiene are: keep your equipment dry and free of antimicrobials; wash your hands often; and store your perishable foods in the refrigerator or freezer. A little dust won't kill you, but a little swipe with a damp sponge might make you sick.

## CHAPTER FOUR

# The Barbarian Bathroom

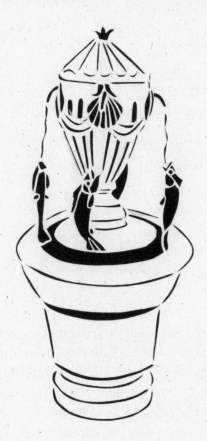

According to the laws of physics, what goes up must come down, and according to the laws of biology, what goes in must come out. For those of us with indoor plumbing, the place where it usually comes out is the bathroom. This concept is apparently quite frightening to many people, who strive to avert the danger posed by bathroom demons by ritually applying poisonous substances to all bathroom surfaces, and saturating the air with fragrant but toxic scents.

**FLUSHED AND FRAGRANT**

The MSDS for a well-known automatic toilet bowl cleaner contains this very specific and detailed list of ingredients:

Chemical

CAS No/Unique ID

Percent

Fragrance(s)/perfume(s)

Dye(s) (unspecified)

Detergent/dispersant additive

Preservative(s) (unspecified)

Sequestrant

I hope this impressively comprehensive list clears up any questions veterinarians or pediatricians may have when they attempt to treat patients who have ingested this product.

Stalwart researchers have discovered that every time a toilet is flushed, microscopic droplets of virus- and bacteria-laden water are launched up to six feet away from the toilet bowl. These teeming droplets may remain aloft for up to seven minutes after the flush.

Solution: Close the lid before you flush.

But what about public toilets, most of which don't sport lids? Dr. Charles Gerba, a microbiologist who has investigated the germ populations in public and private spaces, does not worry about the pathogenic potential of even the most disgusting public toilets. According to Gerba, though it is true that "some viruses can survive for several days to weeks on hard surfaces . . . the germs that you are worried about catching have to get to your nose, mouth, or eyes to infect you." Toilet seat pathogens will not invade via your back-side nor will they migrate up through the soles of your shoes.

So after you use a public toilet, try to refrain from rubbing your eyes, sucking your thumb, chewing your fingernails, or picking your nose until after you have washed your hands.

## FREQUENCY OF FLUSHING

In the last fifty years, the worldwide demand for water has tripled. Water tables are falling due to the overpumping of groundwater. Many inland lakes are shrinking as more and more rivers are being diverted for irrigation and dammed for hydroelectric production, and global warming increases the rate of evaporation. West Africa's Lake Chad has been reduced to 5 percent of its former self; Central Asia's Aral Sea is slowly but surely turning into a salty desert; and the Sea of Galilee is drying up so that mere mortals can occasionally walk where previously only the divine could tread.

While I was writing this chapter, the record-breaking spring flood of 2008 submerged much of Iowa and ruined a large part of its crops, then rolled down the Mississippi River, blowing out levees, inundating small communities, contaminating surface water and groundwater, and permanently polluting wells. In the fields of rural Illinois, the water was ten feet deep and getting deeper all the time. Many of the small towns that were flooded out may never recover and could be permanently abandoned.

Meanwhile, on the West Coast, California's governor, Arnold Schwarzenegger, had to deploy the National Guard to help fight the more than 1,700 forest fires that ignited in February and had burned more than 829,000 acres by July. The fire season usually doesn't reach its peak in California until September. When Governor Schwarzenegger toured the devastation caused by the Humboldt fire, he stated: "[T]he traditional fire season, that went from the end of summer through fall, has extended itself, kind of. Every year the fire season got longer and longer and this year we have seen that there is really no fire season anymore in that sense. The first fires started in February and they go all year through."

Scientists at the Scripps Institution of Oceanography in San Diego analyzed the data from forest fires and found that the number and duration of large wildfires increased "suddenly and dramatically" in the late 1980s. The new and improved 1980s version of the fire season was seventy-eight days longer, and the total area burned was six and a half times larger than it had been a decade earlier. Team member Thomas Swetnam, of the University of Arizona in Tucson, stated, "I see this as one of the first big indicators of climate change impacts in the continental United States. We're showing warming and earlier springs tying in with large forest fire frequencies. Lots of people think climate change and the ecological responses are 50 to 100 years away. But it's not 50 to 100 years away—it's happening now in forest ecosystems through fire."

Whether it is causing drought, fire, or flood, global warming is wreaking havoc with the world's supply of clean drinking water. Fresh, potable water is really too precious to be used to push human waste through sewage pipes. One day the flush toilet will appear ridiculous, and will be as completely outmoded as the slide rule, the button hook, and lead-based paint, but until that day comes, it behooves us to ease up on the flush handle.

## PITHY SAYING

During California's great drought in the late 1970s, witty sages penned this pithy little ditty: "If it's yellow, it's mellow. If it's brown, flush it down." This advice is as pertinent as it ever was, though those of us whose bladders are not what they were in our prechildbearing days may discover that our low-flow toilets need to be flushed after every dozen or so visits—regardless of the color of the contents—in order to prevent our pipes from clogging up with toilet paper.

## BUILDING A BETTER TOILET

According to the experts, the average adult produces between 0.6 and 2.5 liters of urine each day. The average young, healthy, nonpregnant adult has a maximum bladder capacity of approximately one pint; almost everyone else has a smaller holding capacity. Though we hold more, most people feel the urge to empty when their bladders are holding 150 milliliters (ml) of urine, and at the 300 ml mark, we are squirmingly uncomfortable.

Experts inform us that the average person flushes a toilet between seven and nine times each day, and estimate that 75 percent of trips to the bathroom are for urination only. High-flow toilets use up to 6 gallons per flush, while standard low-flow toilets use 1.6 gallons per flush. Though low-flow toilets are a vast improvement over the high-flow models, low-flow toilets still use approximately 6,056 ml of water to flush away 150 to 300 ml of urine.

## PUSH-BUTTON CONVENIENCE

Dual-flush toilets feature a half-flush button that initiates a .8-gallon flush designed to deal with urine, and a full-flush button that sets off a 1.6-gallon flush for solids. The dual-flush toilet is a definite improvement over the standard-flush toilet, but it could be better; the half-flush still sends ten times as much water as urine down the waste pipe. The least expensive dual-flush toilets cost about 75 percent more than the least expensive low-flow toilets, but as the dual-flush toilets become more popular, the price should drop. A variety of reasonably priced dual-flush retrofit kits are available online. The kits are easy to install, and no additional plumbing is necessary to covert your existing toilet into a water-saving paragon.

## NO-MIX

If excessive amounts of nitrogen and phosphorus are released into surface waters, they cause rampant algal growth. When these algal blooms die and begin to rot, they can suck all the oxygen out of the water, killing every living thing that cannot make a hasty retreat.

Although urine makes up only 1 percent of the volume of urban wastewater, it contributes 80 percent of the nitrogen and 50 percent of the phosphorus to the wastewater stream. Removing excess nitrogen and phosphorus at the waste treatment plant is an expensive but necessary process.

Researchers at the Swiss Federal Institute of Aquatic Science and Technology demonstrated that separate collection and treatment of urine could greatly reduce water pollution, reduce the costs of sewage treatment, and last but not least, allow the urine to be easily recycled into fertilizer.

The No-Mix toilet, which the researchers tested at a school and a research institute, has a divided bowl that separates human wastes: liquids go in the front and solids are deposited in the back. Water flushes the solids into the sewer system. Urine is sent into a local storage tank.

The researchers reported that the study's participants had a very positive attitude toward the toilet, despite the fact that one version of the fixture required men to urinate while sitting down.

## WATERLESS URINALS

The waterless urinal seems a more practical tool for recovering usable urine than does the No-Mix toilet.

Conventional urinals use at least three liters (one gallon) of water per flush, while high-tech waterless urinals require neither water nor a flushing system. Waterless urinals are made of specially glazed, perfectly smooth ceramic, or of synthetic materials with a liquid-repelling gel coating. Liquids cannot stick to these surfaces, and neither can odor-causing bacteria—the urine flows off the surfaces of these urinals and is funneled through a trap that contains a biodegradable liquid sealant that is lighter than water. The urine flows right through the sealant and the sealant closes up after it, preventing odors from wafting up from the urinal. A study conducted at the University of California, Santa Barbara, showed that the waterless urinals required half as much maintenance and cleaning as did the conventional, flushing models. Since liquids are only flowing out of, not into, waterless urinals, these fixtures require less plumbing than do the conventional flushing models, so are less expensive to install.

### A Few Varieties of Waterless Urinals

*Cartridge*
Falcon Waterfree Technologies: www.falconwaterfree.com

*Cartridge-Free*
Duravit Architec McDry Waterless Urinal: www.duravit.com
Kohler Waterless: Urinals www.us.kohler.com/onlinecatalog/
    waterless urinal
Waterless No-Flush Urinals: www.waterless.com/ecotrap
ZeroFlush: www.zeroflush.com
Zurn Waterless Urinal: www.zurn.com

Waterless urinals have even been installed at the Taj Mahal, the Rose Bowl Stadium, the Statue of Liberty, and McMurdo Station in Antarctica. If waterless urinals work well for one of the world's most transcendentally beautiful buildings, for beer-soaked sports fans, for Lady Liberty, and for scientists living under the most extreme conditions on earth, they are probably good enough for the average household. A combination of a waterless urinal, a composting toilet, and a gray-water collection system might be just the ticket for the true green householder.

## HUMAN DUNG

After his grand agricultural tour of China in the early twentieth century, F. H. King wrote in his book *Farmers of Forty Centuries*: "[In China] one-sixth of an acre of good land is ample for the maintenance of one person. . . ." In 2007, Cornell researchers determined that, using modern agricultural methods, it takes nearly half an acre of good American cropland to support a vegetarian on a low-fat diet.

Chinese farmers were far more efficient than Western farmers in King's day, and he believed that the difference in crop yields was due to the Chinese habit of composting all organic waste and returning it to the land, and he wrote of Westerners: "Man is the most extravagant accelerator of waste the world has ever endured. His withering blight has fallen upon every living thing within his reach, himself not excepted; and his besom of destruction in the uncontrolled hands of a generation has swept into the sea soil fertility which only centuries of life could accumulate, and yet this fertility is the substratum of all that is living." Dr. King also quoted Dr.

Arthur Stanley, the health officer of the city of Shanghai, who reported in 1899: "The main problem of sanitation is to cleanse the dwelling day by day, and if this can be done at a profit so much the better. While the ultra-civilized Western elaborates destructors for burning garbage at a financial loss and turns sewage into the sea, the Chinaman uses both for manure. He wastes nothing while the sacred duty of agriculture is uppermost in his mind. . . . While to adopt the water-carriage system for sewage and turn it into the river, whence the water supply is derived, would be an act of sanitary suicide."

Composting toilets require a bit more work from their owners than do flushing toilets, but sometime in the near future, if we want to continue to thrive on this small blue-green planet, we will need to begin to compost all our exudates, either in on-site composting toilets, or downstream at municipal sewage treatment plants. In fact, in many areas, farmers' demand for composted municipal biosolids has already outstripped the supply.

## TERMS OF EXCREMENT

My big, antique Webster's dictionary contains the following definitions:

manurance n. 1. Tenure, occupation, or control. Cultivation; tillage; training. Manuring.

manure n. Any material which fertilizes land; a fertilizing substance; specif. refuse of stables and barnyards, consisting of animal excreta with or without litter, the dung of birds, or the like. Cultivation, tillage.

manure v.t. To work with the hand, to cultivate by manual labor. To have in possession; to hold, as land; also, to have in hand, to manage; conduct. To cultivate or till (land); hence, to develop by culture; to cultivate; to train. *Manure thyself then; to thyself be improved. Donne.* To apply manure to; to enrich, as land, by the application of a fertilizing substance. To work up; manipulate; handle; maneuver.

These terms of excrement were certainly also terms of endearment. When the vast majority of people worked the land for a living, the value of manure was quite obvious to them; but now that so many of us are urbanized, we need to work to regain our sense of humus.

## NO-NO'S—SINK, TUB, AND SHOWER DRAINS

When bathroom drains are running sluggishly, chances are good they are clogged with human hair. There are easy steps you can take to decrease the incidence of these clogs. First, reduce the amount of hair going down the drain by installing drain strainers in all your drains. Then remind all residents of the house that hair does not dissolve in water and will not disappear if washed down the drain. Neither will dental floss. Though hair is biodegradable and could, in theory, eventually biodegrade in a drain, dental floss is synthetic and cannot biodegrade. Ever.

Inform hairy, indifferent offenders that if they continue to wash their clumps of shed hair down the drain rather than throwing them in the trash, the next time the drain needs cleaning, the job is theirs. Make them watch as you clean out the drain.

No matter how careful one is, however, into all drains some hair will fall, and eventually that hair will need to be cleaned out.

Chemical drain cleaners contain either very strong sulfuric or hydrochloric acid, or very strong bases such as potassium hydroxide, sodium hypochlorite, or sodium hydroxide. If these corrosive substances are spilled they can start fires, emit toxic fumes, and eat right through any organic object they encounter, including the floor or your foot. When they go down the drain, they adversely affect the bacteria that are necessary to keep a septic tank or sewage treatment plant functioning. It's much better to use a little muscle power to remove obstructions from the plumbing.

The easiest, most nontoxic way to remove hairy obstructions from the drain is to use a handy little drain-cleaning brush that can be found at most hardware stores. This tool looks like a giant pipe cleaner with white nylon bristles and a plastic handle. If you cannot find one of these, you can modify a similar, two-handled brush that is designed to clean behind faucets: Use a wire cutter to sever one of the handles, and you have a perfect drain-cleaning tool.

To use the drain brush, slowly push the small end down the drain, then very, very slowly pull it up. Use your free hand as a shield over the top of the drain brush in order to avoid spattering green slime and bits of hair all over yourself. Pull the bits of gooey hair from the drain brush, and then repeat the operation until you have removed all the hair from the drain. Remove the hair, rinse off the drain brush, and store it under the sink until the next time your drain slows down.

There are also long, thin, toothed, plastic drain cleaners that look rather like demented zippers. These things work well, but are a bit sharp to be safely cleaned off for reuse, and are considered disposable. These zip cleaners are quite narrow and can be stuffed through very small holes.

If your drain is clogged deeper down, please consult my previous book, *Organic Housekeeping* (*Green Housekeeping* for the paperback edition), for complete directions for using a drain snake or a plunger.

## ODOR CONTROL

Life is smelly, life is messy. When your bathroom gets a bit noisome, here's what you can do.

Don't be embarrassed. You are not the only person in the world whose ordure stinks. (My son informs me that he farts nothing but butterflies and lavender, but he always has been exceptional.) The rest of us may benefit from the following information.

Don't use "air fresheners." Adding perfumed petroleum products to your air will not enhance your health, and ill health really stinks. Air fresheners do not clean the air or even remove the offensive smells; they simply fill the air with volatile organic chemicals, some of which overwhelm and desensitize our noses. If the weather permits, open a window. The air will smell better and will actually be cleaner afterward.

Light a match. The flame will consume the odor. But do not throw the match away until after you have quenched it with water—flaming wastebaskets emit unattractive smells. You can also make a more permanent improvement in your bathroom's air quality by installing a humidity-loving plant, a fern for instance, in the bathroom. Unlike synthetic "air fresheners," plants actually improve air quality by consuming carbon dioxide, producing oxygen, and filtering toxins and particulate matter out of the air.

Do not leave damp, dirty laundry moldering in a pile on your bathroom floor or in your bathroom hamper. Mildew smells bad; so do dirty socks.

Fix leaks promptly (see previous remark about mildew).

High humidity encourages the growth of mold and mildew. If the weather permits and your bathroom sports a window, keep the window open while you shower or bathe. If your bathroom is windowless or the weather is uncooperative, turn on the ventilation fan before you turn on the water, and keep the fan going for half an hour after you finish your ablutions.

## FRAGRANCES IN STRANGE PLACES—ROLLING ALONG

There are toilet paper rollers that are loaded with fragrances that possess names such as "Paradise Breeze," "Rainflower Mist," "Simply Vanilla," and "Mountain Fresh." The comic possibilities of such names are nearly endless. Unfortunately, the contents of these products are not so cute. The Material Safety Data Sheet (MSDS) of one prominent brand of scented toilet paper roller shows that the product contains benzyl acetate and concentrated perfume oil. The ingredients that go into fragrances and perfumes are generally considered proprietary information, and the companies that manufacture them are legally allowed to keep their ingredients secret, but the MSDS for benzyl acetate states that the chemical is a skin irritant, an eye irritant, a gastrointestinal tract irritant, may affect the urinary tract, may be toxic to the central nervous system, and is hazardous if ingested or inhaled. Benzyl acetate also causes cell mutations in bacteria, yeasts, and mammals.

I prefer not to subject the most tender part of my anatomy to toilet paper that has been fumigated with chemicals that may irritate the skin and the gastrointestinal and urinary tracts, and are known to induce mutations in yeasts and bacteria.

## BATH LINENS

Bathrooms are frequently humid, and their surfaces are often splashed with water. It behooves any gentleperson who wants to do the minimum of cleaning to reduce the quantity of textiles in the bathroom. Though bath towels, hand towels, washcloths, and bath mats obviously belong in the bathroom, installing wall-to-wall carpeting and putting fuzzy decorative covers on the toilet tank, the lid, and the splash zone immediately in front of the toilet is just asking for trouble. (Of course, if a household includes very young boys, having walls in the bathroom might also be considered a mistake.)

Many mothers nag because they are trying to reduce the amount of cleaning they must do. Doing less cleaning is better for the environment. Reusing everything as many times as possible is one of the best ways to reduce the amount of work one must do. Washing a bath towel after each use is a waste of time, energy, water, and money. Towels are supposed to be used to dry the body after it has already been thoroughly washed and rinsed, and should, theoretically, be clean for at least a week. This theory, however, often breaks down in practice. Half of my family members have been known to emerge from the shower after a long day of gardening, with damp dirt still decorating the backs of their legs, their knees, or their elbows. This damp dirt is then wiped off on a towel. If your towels are frequently besmirched with dirt, and if this dirt stains, you may want to invest in towels that match the color of your indigenous soil. "Natural"-colored cotton towels are also a good choice for those who don't want to have to labor over their bath linens.

If you want to reduce your laundry chores and decrease your water and energy use, remember to wash your entire body, not just the parts that you can see, before you exit the shower, so you can use the same towel for at least a week. Don't leave your damp towel and washcloth on the floor where they will mildew; hang them up.

## USE IT ONE MORE TIME

A towel that has been used to dry off a well-washed adult for a mere week is a large piece of relatively clean, highly absorbent material. By starting with the cleanest surfaces and working toward the dirtiest ones, you can use that towel to dry and polish your mirror, walls, counter, sink, shower stall, and bathroom floor before you throw the limp, bedraggled towel in the laundry hamper.

## SHOWER CURTAIN

The vinyl shower curtain is not only cheap and flimsy, it may also, according to a report released in June 2008 by the Center for Health, Environment, & Justice, hazardous to the user's health. Laboratory tests showed that the "new shower curtain smell" contains up to 108 different volatile organic compounds (VOCs), including high concentrations of toluene, cyclohexanone, methyl isobutyl ketone (MIBK), phenol, and ethylbenzene. VOCs can irritate the eyes, nose, and throat; cause headaches, loss of coordination, and nausea; and can damage the liver, kidneys, and central nervous system. All of the tested shower curtains contained phthalates, which readily migrated to the outer surface of the shower curtain and then evaporated into the air. Some phthalates have been linked to reproductive problems. In addition, all of the tested shower curtains contained one or more of the following dangerous elements: lead, cadmium, mercury, and chromium.

The shower curtains were still emitting some VOCs when the study ended after twenty-eight days. Really cheap vinyl shower curtains may not last much longer than the period of the study.

Solution: Invest in a cotton or nylon shower curtain that can be thrown in the washing machine. We've been using the same sturdy shower curtain for years.

## CLEANING THE HARD SURFACES

The smoother the surface, the easier it is to clean. Bathrooms are full of smooth, shiny surfaces that would be a snap to clean if it weren't for all that water.

There are a few simple things that can be done to reduce bathroom cleaning time.

Keep your shiny surfaces smooth and shiny by avoiding the use of harsh, abrasive cleansers and scrubbers. Fiberglass and acrylic tubs, shower stalls, sinks, and countertop surfaces are relatively soft and easily scratched, and even glazed ceramic will eventually roughen if cleaned too harshly.

The type of soap you are using will greatly affect the amount of soap scum that builds up in your shower, tub, and sink basin. Natural soaps that are made with animal fats (stearic acid) react with the minerals in hard water to produce soap scum. Most commercial bath soaps are actually petroleum-based detergents. These products do not react with the minerals in water and do not form soap scum. If you would rather not clean yourself with a petroleum product, but dislike soap scum, you might want to switch to castile soap, which is made from vegetable oil. Castile soap does not react with the minerals in hard water; its residues never harden and are quite easy to scrub off with just a brush.

Mold and mildew thrive in damp places. Don't allow your bathroom surfaces to remain wet. Vent humid air out of the bathroom and wipe or squeegee down the shower walls after each shower.

When hard water evaporates, it leaves its minerals behind. You can prevent a lot of these mineral deposits by wiping down your sink, counter, and bathtub after each use and either wiping down or squeegeeing your shower stall.

Full-strength white distilled vinegar can be used to clean mineral deposits and hard water spots from many surfaces.

Note: Vinegar dissolves marble and limestone and should never be used on these surfaces. Use a neutral cleaner such as very dilute liquid castile soap instead. Rinse and dry well.

In order to use vinegar to clean a bathroom, fill a spray bottle with white distilled vinegar.

Spray the grubbier surfaces such as the sink bowl, faucets, countertop, bathtub, and shower stall with vinegar. Let it sit for a few minutes and then scrub the grime off with a scrub brush. Rinse the surface with clean water, then wipe it with a clean, dry cloth.

Heavy mineral deposits on plumbing fixtures can be dissolved with a vinegar poultice. Soak a clean cloth in vinegar. Wrap the mineralized faucet in the wet cloth, then wrap the cloth in a plastic bag and secure the plastic with rubber bands or twine. Let it sit overnight, then remove the poultice. Use a scrub brush or old toothbrush to remove the softened deposit. Rinse. (My father-in-law informs me that he used this technique to remove decades-old rust stains in a bathtub. Nothing else he tried had worked.)

Relatively clean surfaces such as mirrors, windows, walls, and the floor can be sprayed and then wiped dry with a clean cloth; vinegar leaves no residue and does not need to be rinsed off.

## TOILET CLEANING

Spray vinegar on the inside of the bowl above the water line. Pour or spray a few tablespoons of vinegar into the bowl. Let it sit for a few minutes, then scrub out the bowl with a toilet brush.

Spray the rest of the toilet with vinegar, and then wipe all the surfaces clean with a small wad of toilet paper. Throw the toilet paper in the bowl.

If the toilet bowl requires heavier cleaning, use a toilet plunger to push as much of the water as possible out of the bowl, then pour a gallon of white distilled vinegar into the toilet bowl. Let it sit overnight while the vinegar softens and dissolves the mineral deposits. The next morning you can use a toilet brush to scrub the softened deposits out of the bowl. The vinegar smell will disappear as soon as the surfaces dry.

## BATTLE-READY

The well-appointed Green Barbarian bathroom is equipped with: bath linens that are color-coordinated with the local earth, so they always look clean; castile soap, which doesn't form soap scum; a spray bottle of vinegar, for quick and easy cleaning; plain, unscented toilet paper, which is easy on the nether parts; a drain brush to keep those drains running freely; and last but not least, a box of matches and a Boston fern, to rid the air of unwanted odors. Tough Green Barbarians choose their hazards carefully; they never succumb to cleaning fumes.

## Chapter Five

# Barbarian Laundry

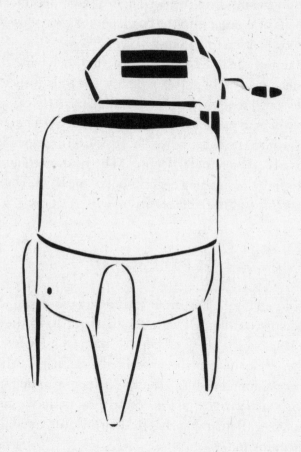

**PRIMITIVE LAUNDRY**

Rivers and streams with conveniently located rocks were the original Laundromats.

## CLASSICAL LAUNDRY

"The washerman launders at the riverbank in the vicinity of the crocodile. . . . His food is mixed with filth, and there is no part of him which is clean. He cleans the clothes of a woman in menstruation. He weeps when he spends all day with a beating stick and a stone there. One says to him, dirty laundry, come to me, the brim overflows."
—From Dua-Khety's advice to his son Pepy, written during the twelfth dynasty of ancient Egypt

The ancient Romans wore woolen dresses in a hot climate, thus their clothing frequently needed a thorough cleaning. The clothes were washed in tubs or vats, and the agitation was supplied by professional cleaning specialists called fullones, who stomped the clothing clean. The alkaline cleaning solution was the urine of men and animals mixed with water. In order to procure enough urine to do their job, the fullones placed large vessels at street corners where male pissersby could contribute to the cleanliness of society. The fullones also scoured the clothing with fuller's earth, a light-colored, refined type of clay that absorbs grease.

After the clothes had been washed, they were rinsed several times, then hung out to dry. The fullones softened the dry clothing by brushing it with teasel (a thistlelike plant that forms very stiff, spiny seed heads). Next, the clothes were spread out flat on a large, loosely woven basket that was set like a dome over the top of a vat of steaming sulfur. The sulfurous steam whitened the clothes and removed stains.

## THE MODERN LAUNDRY ERA

### MONDAY WAS WASHDAY

Before the advent of washing machines, when Monday was the designated day for doing laundry, the chore took up an entire day and required fifty gallons of water per load. Tuesday was ironing day—after the clothes had been boiled, then wrung out by hand, the cotton or linen clothes were so stiff, twisted, wrinkled, and malformed that they could not be worn until they had been ironed smooth.

## LAUNDRY SOAP

In the 1800s, most laundry soap was produced at home by boiling animal fat with wood ashes. Washing clothes by hand with this extremely harsh soap was apt to make the clothes look good while ruining the appearance of the hands.

The first English patent for a washing machine was issued in 1691 for a washing and wringing machine; this invention was followed by many other human-powered washing machines. It seems, however, that a century and a half later, these contraptions were still not in common use. In her 1843 book, *A Treatise on Domestic Economy*, Catharine Beecher neglects to mention washing machines. Here is Beecher's list of laundry-day essentials:

> Two wash-forms are needed; one for the two tubs in which to put the suds, and the other for blueing and starching-tubs. Four tubs, of different sizes, are necessary; also, a large wooden dipper (as metal is apt to rust); two or three pails; a grooved wash-board; a clothes-line (sea-grass, or horse-hair is best); a wash-stick to move clothes, when boiling, and a wooden fork to take them out. Soap-dishes, made to hook on the tubs, save soap and time. Provide, also, a clothes-bag, in which to boil clothes; an indigo-bag, of double flannel; a starch-strainer, of coarse linen; a bottle of ox-gall for calicoes; a supply of starch, neither sour nor musty; several dozens of clothes-pins, which are cleft sticks, used to fasten clothes on the line; a bottle of dissolved gum Arabic; two clothes-baskets; and a brass or copper kettle, for boiling clothes, as iron is apt to rust.

The hand-cranked wringer-washer was invented in 1861; then, in the early 1900s, adding an electric or gasoline motor to a wringer-washer became an option. Many people who had once washed their clothes by hand in a washtub became so fond of these efficient machines, which required only forty gallons of water per load, that they continued to use their old wringer-washers until the 1960s, long after most other Americans had switched to automatic electric washing machines. The Amish still use wringer-washers.

## MODERN WASHING MACHINES

Traditional automatic washing machines use an average of forty-one gallons of water per load, while in order to be classified as "high efficiency," washing machines must use less than twenty-seven gallons of water per load. This means that even the least efficient washing machine is more energy- and water-efficient than hand laundering. My highly efficient Swedish ASKO washing machine uses between 5.7 and 9 gallons of water per load, which is a good thing, because our well is quite shallow and slow. (My son points out that I am very smug about my washing machine. It is certainly true that I am quite fond of it. It is also true that during a prolonged dry spell a few years ago, our well would certainly have run dry if we had been using a standard washing machine. That drought forced a few of our neighbors to drill new wells.)

Front-loading washing machines are more energy- and water-efficient than top loaders. The tumbling action of front loaders also cleans clothes more gently than does the agitator of a top loader. Even though front loaders can be more expensive than top loaders, the savings in energy, detergent, and wear and tear on clothing may make up for the larger initial cost of a more efficient machine.

If you have access to a modern, automatic washing machine, thank your lucky stars, throw in a load of laundry, then go out and enjoy your free time! If you use your washing machine at night, when the demand for electricity is generally the lowest, your laundering activities will have the lowest possible environmental impact. (Power plants must run continuously, when electrical demand is high, and more fuel is used to produce more electricity, but during "off-peak hours" the demand for electricity may be met by the power plant's "idle" setting.)

## CLOTHES DRYERS VS. CLOTHESLINES

Electric dryers account for between 5 and 10 percent of the residential electricity use in the United States. Drying clothes on the line may save a householder more than $100 in electricity each year.

Whenever the weather permits, do yourself and the environment a favor and hang that laundry out to dry. If you smooth out your clothes and hang them with care, they will end up sweet-smelling and relatively wrinkle-free.

Hanging clothes up to dry indoors works well if the weather is dry, but in extremely humid weather when the furniture, walls, and people are all sweating, wet laundry hung up indoors may mildew before it dries out.

## THE HOA (HOME OWNERS' ASSOCIATION) VS. THE CLOTHESLINE

The Community Associations Institute estimates that there are 300,000 homeowner and condominium cooperatives in the United States, and one out of every five Americans lives under the aegis of an HOA.

These HOAs can, and sometimes do, dictate almost every visible aspect of their residents' domestic lives, in order to maintain property values. If you go online and peruse any random HOA's Declaration of Covenants, Conditions, and Restrictions, you are likely to find rules dictating the allowable colors of house paint; roof type and color (these rules are frequently invoked to prevent residents from installing solar panels); height and style of buildings, including outbuildings; and allowable colors of "window treatments." The covenants also dictate landscaping styles and plants; lawn height (short), color (green), and size (large); permissible fence styles, materials, and colors; whether or not visible antennas, satellite dishes, boats, or recreational vehicles are allowed; style of welcome mats; the maximum number of overnight visitors; whether or not residents are allowed to use clotheslines; and last but not least, whether residents can fly the American flag from a flagpole (usually not).

Unfortunately, these HOA covenants are legally binding. The board members of many HOAs have the power to levy fines for noncompliance, and can make special assessments for neighborhood capital improvements.

HOA boards can and do foreclose on the homes of homeowners who do not pay their assessments, HOA dues, or fines on time.

## DIRTY LITTLE SECRETS

In the summer of 2007, Susan Taylor, a resident of Awbrey Butte, an exclusive neighborhood in Oregon, decided to help reduce her impact on the environment by drying her clothes outdoors on a line. This action violated the Covenants, Conditions, and Restrictions of Awbrey Butte's HOA, which requires that "clothes drying apparatus . . . shall be screened from view." Unfortunately, fencing is explicitly discouraged in Awbrey Butte's covenants.

Within a few days Ms. Taylor began getting complaints, including one from the subdivision's developer, which warned, "laundry lines are not permitted in the Awbrey Butte Subdivision," and added, "many owners in Awbrey Butte take great pride in their home and surrounding areas." Ms. Taylor responded with a letter in which she asserted that the rule is "outdated" because of the risk posed by global warming. The HOA replied with a letter stating that Ms. Taylor must "discontinue this practice by July 9, 2007, to avoid legal action which will be taken after that date." The article quoted a neighbor's opinion about the clothesline: "This bombards the senses. It can't possibly increase property values and make people think this is a nice neighborhood."

These controlled neighborhoods are definitely "nice," according to the original meaning of the word: "Exacting in matters of taste; fastidious; in a derogatory sense, over dainty, finical . . ."As Bertrand Russell wrote in his essay "Nice People," "The chief characteristic of nice people is the laudable practice of improvement upon reality. God made the world, but nice people feel that they could have done the job better."

## ELEGANT CLOTHESLINES

My husband and I gardened for many years for a woman who lived on a large estate in Duluth. Her big, handsome, three-story brick-and-stone mansion was built in 1916 and sported stone and wood carvings, stained and leaded glass, and a couple of acres of lovely gardens. The grounds also featured a neat, brick-paved laundry yard that was nestled behind high brick walls that bristled with hooks for clotheslines. On hot, sunny days, the laundry yard got very hot and must have baked the laundry dry quite quickly.

## DRYING EQUIPMENT

There are many varieties of clotheslines, drying racks, and accessories, and some of these are elegantly engineered.

Retractable clotheslines can be used indoors or outdoors, and allow the user to get the clothesline out of the way when it is not in use. Many retractable clothesline units feature multiple lines.

Rigid drying racks that can be folded down and placed out of the way when their services are not required are commonly used indoors by the frilly-lingerie set. These are also quite useful for drying socks, mittens, and other outdoor clothing during rainy or snowy weather.

Sweaters retain their shape better when they are dried flat—a mesh sweater-drying rack provides the perfect surface for this drying job.

A set of pants stretchers consists of a pair of rustproof metal frames that are designed to fit inside pant legs. In order to use pant stretchers, you slide a frame inside a wet pant leg, line the frame up with the crease, and then adjust the frame so it fits tightly inside the pant leg. Repeat with the other pant leg, then hang the pants up to dry. The pants will dry smooth, wrinkle-free, and with a perfect knife-edge crease. I am still anxiously awaiting the invention of the shirt stretcher.

Rotary or umbrella clotheslines resemble square patio umbrellas with rows of clotheslines stretched across the ribs. The shaft of this contraption spins in a socket that is sunk into the ground, and the whole thing can be either folded like an umbrella or lifted out of the ground and stored elsewhere. An umbrella clothesline that is about four feet on a side holds about sixty feet of clothesline.

Pulley clotheslines have two pulleys, each attached to a support. The ends of the clothesline are tied together, and the line runs in a continuous loop supported by the pulleys. This is the classic city clothesline that can run from one building to another and can be used by a person standing on a fire escape, balcony, or at an open window. Clotheslines and clothesline systems can be purchased at hardware stores or online.

Here are a few online vendors that sell drying racks, clotheslines, and accessories:

Lehman's: www.lehmans.com
Vermont Country Store: www.vermontcountrystore.com
Breezecatcher Clothes Dryers: www.breezecatcher.com
Urban Clothes Lines: www.urbanclotheslines.com
Breeze Dryer: www.breezedryer.com

## CLOTHESLINE SEMAPHORE

"Clothes are important status symbols," wrote Ronald G. Klietsch, Ph.D., in a 1969 article entitled "Clothesline Patterns and Covert Behavior." Klietsch was the senior operations research analyst for 3M Company in St. Paul, Minnesota. He continued, "The family wash, collectively speaking, represents a total family presentation. Hence, the family wash may be seen as a set of symbols . . . the 'public' display of the wash involves an 'invisible' audience of neighbors and passers-by whose reactions are essential to the family's identity and the maintenance of their image. . . . The husband's occupational prestige rating, home-ownership, and ownership of an indoor dryer do significantly distinguish among housewives with covert and non-covert clothesline patterns."

Why would a senior operations research analyst for 3M Company be researching housewives' clothes drying habits in 1969? Line-dried clothes naturally tend to be less wrinkled than clothes that have been machine-dried, so permanent-press fabrics and clothes dryers rather neatly complement each other. Unfortunately, the first permanent-press fabrics had a rather serious drawback—they tended to attract and hold oily stains—so 3M modified its Scotchgard fabric finish. The newly formulated Scotchgard helped make permanent press fabrics repel stains and then release them easily when washed. The product was ready, but perhaps the customers needed to be convinced to buy a few more clothes dryers.

However, 3M stopped manufacturing the original Scotchgard, as well as all its other slippery perfluorinated (PFOS) products, in 2000, after research had shown that these chemicals, which are apparently deathless and never biodegrade, had been building up in the environment and bioaccumulating in mammals since the first perfluorinated chemical was invented in 1938. Exposure to PFOSs can induce permanent wrinkles such as birth defects, liver damage, and cancer.

## MODERN LAUNDRY PRODUCTS

Old-fashioned, animal-fat-and-lye laundry soap, like other animal fat–based soaps, reacts with the minerals in hard water to form soap scum. Synthetic laundry detergents, which have almost completely replaced laundry soap, were specifically designed to rinse out completely, leaving no residue behind. Fabric softeners were introduced in the 1950s, shortly after synthetic detergents became popular, because these detergents stripped all the natural oils out of fabrics, leaving the clothes stiff, scratchy, and fully loaded with negative ions that caused static cling. Fabric softeners made the fabric "fluffy" by coating it with fatty compounds and with positively charged surfactants that offset the negative charge that causes static. But all these coating agents made fabric appear dingy. Next the manufacturers invented fluorescent whitening agents, or optical brighteners; these additives give fabrics a "fresh" appearance by converting ultraviolet light into visible blue light, making the fabrics appear blue-white.

All this glowing pulchritude has an environmental cost. Invisible fluorescent dyes commonly contain:

Derivatives of coumarin, which, according to the Material Safety Data Sheet (MSDS), is extremely hazardous if ingested, hazardous if inhaled, is a skin and eye irritant, and is classed as a possible human carcinogen.

Diaminostilbene, which, according to the MSDS, is believed to be toxic if ingested.

Benzidines: Benzidine dihydrochloride is classified as very hazardous if ingested or inhaled, hazardous in case of skin contact, an
eye irritant, and a proven carcinogen. Benzidine dihydrochloride
biodegrades into an even more hazardous substance—3,3'-diamino-
benzidine—which is hazardous if inhaled and may be toxic to the
kidneys, lungs, bladder, upper respiratory tract, skin, and central
nervous system.

A 1960s report by the Geigy Chemical Corporation stated: "Optical
brighteners are needed to increase the total spectral radiance, which normally results in better whiteness and an impression of superior cleanliness."
If your bright-white clothes are permeated with irritating and health-endan-
gering chemicals, are they really clean?

## JAMBALAYA—
### WHITER THAN WHITE, BRIGHTER THAN BRIGHT

Eugene Cioffi, of the University of South Alabama, discovered that fluorescent whitening agents (FWAs) can be used to ascertain whether the
bacteria that are contaminating shellfish beds are of animal or human origin. According to Cioffi's 2004 report, "Detergents are used in very large
quantities, and contribute a significant portion of the load of anthropogenic
chemicals to the aquatic environment." Cioffi stated that after the wash
cycle, 5 to 80 percent of FWAs remain in the washwater and are discharged
into the wastewater stream, and "In general, FWAs do not readily break
down in the environment, remaining either in solution or slowly adsorbing
onto sediment particles." Thus: "The recovery and identification of FWAs
in the Mobile Bay watershed is selectively indicative of human anthropogenic activity."

Bacteria are mortal and transient, but apparently fluorescent whitening
agents are forever.

Dr. Cioffi should be given an award for the most creative and beneficial
use of a persistent pollutant.

## BLENDING IN

There are some situations in which glowing in the dark would be a very, very bad thing.

The laundering instructions for the U.S. Air Force's Airman Battle Uniform (ABU) warn against the use of detergents that contain optical brighteners. The air force found that optical brighteners make the ABU more easily detectable by night vision equipment and also make the uniforms more visible in low-light environments of all kinds, because the chemicals reflect more of the available light. According to the air force, most commercial detergents contain optical brighteners, and it is impossible to ascertain by reading the label whether or not the product contains these fluorescent chemicals.

## NATURALLY SOFT

So how did Great-Grandma make her laundry clean, soft, white, sweet-smelling, and static-free? She used real laundry soap, which contains fatty acids—soap residue acts like a fabric softener. Then, when the laundry was clean, she hung it up to dry in the sun.

## GREENER, CLEANER LAUNDRY

Detergents that do not contain optical brighteners also tend to have fewer chemicals that can damage human and environmental health, such as petroleum distillates, alkylphenol ethoxylates (persistent organic pollutants that disrupt the endocrine system), sodium hypochlorite (chlorine bleach), phosphates (water pollutants), and fragrances. Check the label to make sure.

There are even a couple of detergent alternatives that are gentler on the environment than even the most eco-friendly mineral or plant-based detergents.

The first alternative is good old laundry soap, which seems to have gone completely extinct in the United States. Laundry soap flakes are still being made in Europe, however.

L'Amande Laundry Soap Flakes are tiny bits of a pure vegetable oil–based soap. The flakes are fragrance-free and contain no additives; they give laundry a nice, fresh smell and soft feel.

The Air Force Uniform and Recognition Programs page lists the following detergents as free of optical brighteners and safe for use with the ABU:

All Detergent Free Clear

Allens Laundry Detergent (powder and liquid)

Bi-O-Kleen Laundry Detergent (powder and liquid)

Charlie's Soap (powder and liquid)

Cheer (liquid and powder) Note: This is a scented product. Sending olfactory signals to the enemy may not be a good idea either.

Cheer Free

Country Save Liquid Detergent

ECOS Free and Clear Laundry Detergent

Exchange Select Cold Water Wash

Mountain Green Liquid Laundry Detergent

Nature Clean (liquid and powder)

Oxy-Prime Powder

Planet Ultra (liquid and powder)

Seventh Generation Laundry detergents

Sport-Wash

Sun & Earth Liquid

Surf Powder (not Surf Liquid)

WashEZE

Woolite, original and dark

L'Amande soap flakes are made in Italy, and are readily available online. It may be worth ordering them just for the adorable illustration on the box. The instructions are in Italian. Translated, they read: "To wash by hand: use 1 pugno (handful) of flakes for every 5 liters of water, wash and then rinse. To wash in a machine, use 2 pugni (handfuls) of flakes.

We advise that you consult the instruction manual for instructions for your machine."

I use two heaping tablespoons of these light, fluffy flakes per load of wash in my very efficient front-loading machine. If your machine is a top-loader, you will probably have to use two pugni per load.

Dri-Pak Soap Flakes are manufactured in England from palm and coco-nut oils and contain no additives or fragrances. The Dri-Pak company also used to manufacture Lux Soap Flakes, but Unilever withdrew Lux from the market in 2002. Dri-Pak Soap Flakes are easily available online.

Note: Flame-resistant clothing such as children's sleepwear should not be washed in soap; soap residue impairs the effectiveness of the flame-resistant finishes.

## SOAP THAT GROWS ON TREES

The second, and much more exotic, alternative to detergent is the soap nut, which actually does grow on trees. Soap nut trees (*Sapindus* species) are native to tropical regions, and people have been using the saponin-rich dried fruits of these trees for cleaning purposes for centuries. (Saponins are sugar derivatives that produce a soapy lather when mixed with water.) Com-mercial soap nut plantations are found mostly in India and Nepal. The trees take nine years to begin bearing fruit, but can continue producing until they are a hundred years old.

Soap nuts can be ordered online. They are sold in either whole or pow-dered form.

In order to wash a load with whole soap nuts, one must first enclose three or four soap nuts in a cloth bag or tied-off sock. The water and agita-tion of the wash cycle will release saponins from the soap nuts, though hot water is best because it extracts the saponins more efficiently than warm or cold water. This means that the soap nuts will still be releasing saponins into the rinse water, so your laundry may retain quite a bit of soap nut residue. The soap nuts can be used to wash a couple of loads of wash, and can then be composted.

I have tested soap nuts in both whole and powdered form, and have had much better luck washing my laundry with the powdered soap nuts. Because soap nut powder may clog the filters of a washing machine, and the saponins are released into hot water more easily than into cold water, I boil powdered soap nuts to make soap nut tea.

## MAKING AND USING SOAP NUT TEA

Boil four tablespoons of soap nut powder in one cup of water. Turn off the heat. Allow the tea to cool and then strain out the solids. (A coffee press works very well for straining out the solids.) Store the soap nut tea in a plastic squeeze bottle.

I use about one and a half teaspoons (yes, teaspoons!) of soap nut tea to wash a load of laundry in my front-loading machine; it takes one table-spoon of mineral-based detergent to wash a load of laundry. My washing machine uses a maximum of nine gallons of water per load, so if you have an old, inefficient top loader that uses forty-two gallons of water per load, you would probably need to use nearly three tablespoons of soap nut tea per load.

I have used soap nut tea in hot, cold, and lukewarm washloads. I have washed loads of laundry that included reeking, stinking socks (mine), and everything has come out smelling fresh and clean. This is in stark contrast to what often happens when laundry loads that include my socks are washed in regular detergent—even after a long, hot wash cycle, my socks often emerge still smelling like Limburger. If I'm really unlucky, some of the other items have picked up the smell, too. Soap nut tea is also better at washing all the grease and smell out of washloads of my greasy dishcloths and kitchen tow-els, and all the fish smell out of my husband's work clothes.

I have extremely sensitive skin that overreacts to many detergents, but I have had no trouble at all with soap nuts. In fact, last winter after I fin-ished cutting up our old Christmas tree and hauled its remains outside, I realized that I had smeared dark, sticky sap all over my forearms. Normally I use either cooking oil or citrus solvent to remove pine sap, but this time I decided to try a little full-strength soap nut tea. The sap slid easily off my arms, and my skin did not react to the soap nut tea at all.

Though I have had excellent results using soap nut tea to wash clothes in our mineral-rich well water, I have had reports from other people who have not been impressed by it. If you are interested in using soap nuts, you may need to try them out and see how well you like them. And remember that soap nuts take the place of plain detergent; they do not act as a stain remover or a bleach.

Soap nut powder is available online from Neem Resource: www.neem resource.com; and Nature with Love: www.fromnaturewithlove.com/soap/ product. Whole soap nuts are available from Maggie's Pure Land: www .maggiespureland.com.

## DRY AND DANGEROUS

My paternal grandmother took in dry cleaning for a living; gasoline was the dry-cleaning solvent of choice in the early twentieth century, and the whole family took turns powering the hand-cranked dry-cleaning machine that stood in their backyard. The brain-damaging effects of prolonged exposure to gasoline and gasoline fumes were unknown in that era.

My father and aunt both had serious short-term memory deficits, as do my daughter and I. For many years I had been puzzled by this, but assumed that my memory deficits and my father's gasoline exposure were unrelated, because classical genetics stated that parents can only pass along genetic damage if the genetic code has mutated. Actual genetic mutations do not occur readily unless the subject has been exposed to radioactivity.

Then I read about the developing field of epigenetics, which deals with the inherited effects of exposure to toxins. Scientists have now demonstrated that toxins can change the expression of genes, turning them either on or off, and when parents are exposed to toxins that turn specific genes on or off, these changes can be passed along to their offspring. So it turns out that my father's gasoline exposure could indeed have caused my memory deficits.

Though dry cleaning is no longer as potentially explosive an occupation as it was in the era of petroleum-based dry-cleaning solvents, the modern dry-cleaning solvent, perchloroethylene, is not appreciably less toxic than the solvents that it replaced. Perchloroethylene has many aliases, including perchlor, tetrachloroethylene, ethylene, tetrachloride, carbon dichloride, and "perc." But perchloroethylene by any other name is still dangerous. One thousand out of every 100,000 dry-cleaning workers develops cancer, most commonly cancer of the bladder, kidney, or intestines. This rate is much higher than that of the general population: In 2004, the overall incidence of cancer was 537.6 per 100,000 American males, and 403.1 per 100,000 American females.

A study conducted by the Environmental Protection Agency (EPA) showed that living in the same building as a dry-cleaning establishment poses a health risk. This residential exposure to dry cleaning fumes increases the residents' chances of developing cancer to either one in a hundred or one in a million, depending upon the type of dry-cleaning equipment that is being used. The EPA considers a one-in-a-million chance of developing cancer worth worrying about.

In 1996, researchers from Consumers Union measured the amount of perchlorethylene fumes emanating from freshly dry-cleaned clothing, and estimated that wearing a freshly dry-cleaned blazer and blouse once a week for forty years would give the wearer a 1 in 6,700 risk of developing a cancer that was caused by perc exposure.

No matter how pristine it looks, I don't think that a carcinogenic blouse should be considered clean. Consumers Union recommends that conventional dry cleaning should only be utilized as a last resort, and states that before they are worn, newly dry-cleaned garments should be aired outdoors or in an open garage or outbuilding.

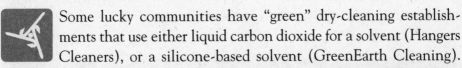 Some lucky communities have "green" dry-cleaning establishments that use either liquid carbon dioxide for a solvent (Hangers Cleaners), or a silicone-based solvent (GreenEarth Cleaning). Consumers Union compared both of these methods to the standard perc dry cleaning and to "wet cleaning," which uses very small amounts of water. The researchers found that the liquid carbon dioxide was the most effective as well as the least damaging method of dry cleaning; the silicone-based method came in second, and the standard perc-based dry cleaning and the "wet" cleaning tied for last place.

A "Dry Clean Only" label indicates that the clothing manufacturer considers the garment too delicate to be cleaned in a washing machine. For instance, handmade lace and some types of rayon are too fragile to withstand machine agitation, and most wool will shrink if subjected to strenuous machine washing and drying. But some garments are labeled "Dry Clean Only" because of cheap and shoddy construction methods that make the items likely to shrink, fray, or change color if washed in water.

If you would rather avoid dry cleaning altogether, read clothing labels before you buy, and try to avoid purchasing items that must be dry cleaned. Some fancy new clothes dryers feature steam-cleaning cabinets wherein even delicate items can be successfully steam cleaned.

For detailed information and instructions about cleaning specific fabrics, and explicit information on dealing with different types of stains, please consult my previous book, *Organic Housekeeping* (*Green Housekeeping* in paperback).

## GET IN, GET CLEAN, GET OUT

Modern laundering should be a safer, easier activity than it was when crocodiles stalked unlucky washermen on the banks of the Nile. Hence, the Green Barbarian laundry is designed to clean clothing while using a minimum of resources and causing a minimum of pollution. Water- and energy-efficient appliances are de rigueur, as are unscented detergents and laundry soaps. And no true Green Barbarian would be caught dead in a freshly dry-cleaned suit, because who really wants to die for a clean suit?

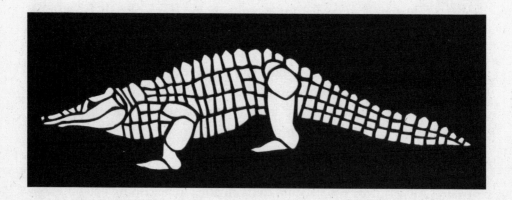

## CHAPTER SIX

# Barbarically Healthy

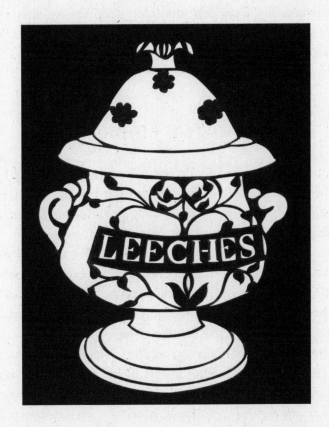

Disclaimer: Please remember that I am not a doctor and that my suggestions are based on my own experiences and reading. Many of the ideas I discuss below are matters of some controversy, and what works for some people may not work for others. Before you start or stop taking any medication or adopt any alternative remedies or treatments, I strongly urge you to consult your own health professional.

## MEMENTO MORI

I have been reading medical studies for some time now, and I hate to be the bearer of bad news, but all the research suggests that humans are mortal, and all of us will eventually die of something. If you concentrate too hard on your health, other things that are actually more important to your quality of life may elude you. If you concentrate solely on your cardiac health, you are pretty likely to shift your greatest risk of death or disability to some other part of your anatomy.

Live bravely!

## DRUGS AND CHEMICALS

Sewage treatment plants and septic systems cannot biodegrade prescription drugs or antimicrobials. Many drugs pass right through sewage treatment plants and end up polluting our waterways, so you should never flush drugs or chemicals down the toilet or pour drugs down the drain.

In order to dispose of drugs safely, either bring them to your hazardous waste facility, or remove the labels from your bottles of defunct drugs, and pour salt and water into the bottle in order to ruin the contents. Then securely cap the bottle, tape the cap on securely, put the bottle in a paper bag, tape it shut, and throw the whole package in the trash.

Unfortunately, though many people are in desperate need of prescription drugs that they cannot afford, it is illegal for private citizens in the United States to "recycle" unused drugs by giving them to people who need them. In some states, and in Canada, nursing homes can recycle prescription drugs after their original owners have passed away if the drugs are still in sealed bottles or blister packs. This is certainly a step in the right direction.

## DISEASE-MONGERING

Pharmaceutical companies, like all other companies, are interested in selling their products. Unfortunately for Big Pharma, a large percentage of their products are aimed at sick people, who are usually outnumbered by those who are healthy. One of the easiest ways to increase the market for pharmaceuticals is to convince people that they are sick. Toward that end, the pharmaceutical industry has been redefining many perfectly normal human states as illnesses. The strategy has been quite successful at turning many healthy human beings into valetudinarians. Medicating ourselves into oblivion (and perhaps into insolvency) will not change the fact that life is sometimes painful, uncomfortable, sad, or jittery.

## INSOMNIA

Americans spend $4.5 billion per year on sleeping pills, but laboratory measurements show that they are far less effective than people think they are.

A single pill of Rozerem, one of the new generation of sleeping pills, will set you back about $3.50 and, according to a study by the National Institutes of Health (NIH), will only buy you an extra eleven minutes of sleep. The NIH study showed that the new generation of sleeping pills work better than placebos, but not much better. Subjects who took older, less expensive drugs such as Halcion and Restoril gained an extra thirty-two minutes of sleep.

People typically overestimated by about twenty minutes how much extra sleep they had gained by taking a sleeping pill. Sleeping pills apparently reduce anxiety and can keep people from worrying about not sleeping, so they feel better. The pills also induce amnesia, which means that people don't remember that they were tossing and turning all night—nor, in the case of Ambien users, do they remember that they were sleepwalking, sleep eating, or sleep driving. A survey of forensic laboratories showed that in some states, Ambien is among the top ten drugs found in the bloodstreams of drivers who are pulled over for impaired driving.

Be brave. A little bit of sleeplessness will not hurt you, and worrying about it will only make it worse. Sleeping pills may induce or aggravate sleep apnea (which can kill you). Sleep driving can kill you. If you have an understanding, willing bedpartner, there are quite a few things you can do in the middle of the night without having to get out of bed.

## RESTLESS LEG SYNDROME

I have been an impressively active sleeper ever since I can remember. I fell out of bed every night when I was a small child, and would spend the rest of the night sleeping peacefully on the floor.

As I got older, the twitchy restlessness acquired a name: restless leg syndrome (RLS). While researching this book, I learned that overly athletic sleeping also has a name: periodic limb movement disorder (PLMD). PLMD is what propelled me out of bed as a child, and what makes my legs kick violently every time I fall asleep after a festive evening of eating what I shouldn't.

After a series of experiments I conducted on myself in my twenties, I gradually figured out what set me off: extreme boredom; sitting too long; not enough exercise; too much exercise; drinking caffeinated beverages in the evening; or eating ice cream before bed. Consequently, I try to get enough exercise; avoid attending boring events; avoid sitting for long periods of time; and I never, ever eat ice cream in the evening. (My sister, who also has restless leg syndrome, cannot eat any chocolate in the evening.)

A year or so ago I was astonished when a television commercial informed me that restless leg syndrome had been declared a neurological disorder that needed to be treated with medication. I could not help admiring the commercial—those advertisers were certainly adept at pushing all the buttons of people with RLS, as they called it.

According to the National Institutes of Health, up to 10 percent of the U.S. population has those itchy, pulling, creepy-crawly, tugging feelings that make them feel as if they will lose their collective mind if they don't move their legs. Apparently the pharmaceutical industry could not resist such a large potential market. When they discovered that a Parkinson's disease drug called ropinirole—brand name Requip—was effective against RLS, they expanded their marketing efforts. Other drugs that may help reduce RLS symptoms include opioids such as codeine or oxycodone, sleeping pills, or anticonvulsants. Unfortunately, all of these drugs have side effects. Requip may induce compulsive eating, compulsive shopping, gambling addiction, sexual addiction, or other addictive behaviors. Requip's less amusing side effects include dizziness, nausea, and fainting. Opioids are addictive and may cause dizziness, nausea, and vomiting. Anticonvulsants can cause dizziness, fatigue, and insomnia.

According to the National Institutes of Health, healthy people who suffer from restless leg syndrome may be able to fend off the creepy-crawlies by getting moderate exercise, maintaining a regular sleeping schedule, and decreasing the use of caffeine, alcohol, and tobacco. Or they can continue to overeat, avoid exercise, keep smoking, drink coffee and booze at night, and medicate themselves with Requip, a drug that may make them lose their shirt at the casino, spend all their money at the mall, eat themselves into a stupor, or try to mate with anything that slows down.

## ONE PILL, TWO PILLS, RED PILL, BLUE PILL

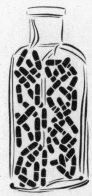

"The art of medicine consists in amusing the patient while nature cures the disease."

—Voltaire

The history of the placebo is a long, noble, and continuous one. The ancient Egyptians, Greeks, Romans, and Chinese all used treatments and concoctions that had no active pharmacological ingredients but were nevertheless often effective.

Studies have shown that the color of a placebo pill influences patients' reactions. For example, red placebos are more effective at relieving pain than are white, blue, or green placebos. Yellow pills are better for treating depression than are white pills. Two placebo pills are better than one, no matter what they are supposed to be treating. When volunteers are given placebo pills but no information about their expected effects, blue pills tranquilize, while red pills act as stimulants. Subjects fall asleep more quickly after taking a blue capsule than after taking an orange capsule.

A study published in March 2008 by behavioral economist Dan Ariely showed that placebo pills work better when they cost more. Eighty-two volunteers were told that they were testing a new painkiller. Half the subjects were told the painkiller cost $2.50 per dose, while the rest of the subjects were told that the dose had been marked down to ten cents because the pills had been bought in bulk for the test. The volunteers were given light electric shocks before and after they took the pills. Eighty-five percent of the subjects who thought they had ingested a $2.50 pill said they felt less pain from the electrical shock after taking the pill, while 61 percent of those who thought they had ingested a ten-cent pill thought they felt less pain because of the pill.

Bear in mind that these placebo pills contained no active ingredients of any kind. Perhaps the next time I have a headache I should just swallow an expensive red jellybean.

Or maybe I should hum. . . .

## JUST HUMMING ALONG

An estimated 14 percent of the American populace suffers from chronic sinusitis, which can block the nasal passages, blunt the sense of smell, and cause breathing difficulties, headache, sore throat, coughing, sinus infection, and tooth pain. Severe sinusitis can even cause nasal polyps.

Swedish researchers have discovered that humming causes a 92 percent increase in the flow of air between the sinuses and the nose. Along with the increased airflow comes an increase in the levels of nitric oxide in the nasal passages. Nitric oxide is produced in the sinuses and is part of the body's defense against invading microorganisms.

According to a congested researcher in Texas, humming in low tones produces the strongest vibrations. Clearing badly clogged sinuses may require long humming sessions of 60 to 120 hums per hour, up to four times a day. Humming may also help relieve the symptoms of the common cold. But the researcher cautioned against humming while driving, because intense humming may induce dizziness.

Researchers have also found that meditation increases the amount of nitric oxide in the bloodstream. Perhaps humming can induce more than dizziness . . . *ommmmm*. . . .

My husband, who has chronically blocked sinuses, perhaps because of the dustiness of his job, tried out the humming technique. He found that it did help him breathe more easily. He even tried humming on a kazoo, but found that kazoo-induced vibrations didn't reach his sinuses. We were profoundly disappointed that kazooing didn't rattle his sinuses, because we were contemplating founding a new religion whose practitioners would march around tooting on kazoos in order to reach Nirvana. I can't sit still, but I can hum.

## GET UP, STAND UP

A study published in 2007 by scientists at the University of Missouri, Columbia, demonstrated that going to the gym for an hour every day is not likely to make people healthy if they are inactive during the rest of their waking hours.

Marc Hamilton, an associate professor of biomedical sciences, led the team that studied the impact of inactivity on rats, pigs, and humans. They found evidence that all the research subjects, no matter how furry they were or how many feet they had, were adversely affected by long periods of sitting, and exercising for an hour a day was not enough to reverse the effect. According to Hamilton: "The enzymes in blood vessels of muscles responsible for 'fat burning' are shut off within hours of not standing. Standing and moving lightly will re-engage the enzymes, but since people are awake 16 hours a day, it stands to reason that when people sit much of that time they are losing the opportunity for optimal metabolism throughout the day."

Apparently, standing uses twice as much energy as sitting. The scientists recommend that people stand up as much as possible during the day because, according to Hamilton: "There is a large amount of energy associated with standing every day that can't be easily compensated for by thirty to sixty minutes at the gym."

And researchers at the Mayo Clinic in Rochester, Minnesota, found that people's "nonexercise activity thermogenesis," or NEAT, determines who is lean and who is obese. These researchers found that obese people, on average, sit 150 minutes longer each day than their slender counterparts. This extra sitting conserves an extra 350 calories per day, which can then be conveniently stored as fat. According to James Levine, M.D., "A person can expend calories either by going to the gym, or through everyday activities. Our study shows that the calories that people burn in their everyday activities—their NEAT—are far, far more important in obesity than we previously imagined."

The study involved, among other things, customized, data-logging underwear that could monitor the body positions and movements of the ten obese people and ten lean people who volunteered for the study. The results showed that it is metabolically more effective to put more NEAT into your life in order to be healthy than it is to pursue organized exercise. Officially sanctioned NEAT activities include standing, pacing, twitching, fidgeting, drumming on tabletops, gesticulating while talking, foot tapping, hair twiddling, and last but not least, gum chewing, which, if you chew a really big wad, burns up eleven calories per hour.

Lean and annoying. That's our motto!

## UNBUTTERED

In December 2007, the Centers for Disease Control and Prevention announced that the average cholesterol levels of American adults dropped to 199 in 2006. This was the first time in almost fifty years that the average cholesterol levels had fallen within the recommended range. According to the report, the percentage of American adults with high cholesterol (defined as levels of 240 mg per dl of blood or higher) decreased to 16 percent in 2006, down from 20 percent in the early 1990s. Experts attribute the decrease in cholesterol levels to the increased use of anticholesterol medications. In 2006, more than 4 percent of Americans ages twenty to forty-four were taking cholesterol-lowering drugs, as were more than a quarter of all Americans ages sixty-five and older.

A study published in the *European Journal of Epidemiology* in 2000 that compared the blood cholesterol levels of Americans and Germans found that the average cholesterol levels in the Federal Republic of Germany were more than twenty points higher than those in the United States, yet Germans are less likely to die of coronary heart disease than are Americans. (In 2000, the average German male's cholesterol was 240 versus the average American male's 218. The average German female's cholesterol was 248 versus the American female's 225.)

Indo-Asians have the highest incidence of coronary artery disease in the world, despite the fact that nearly half of them are lifelong vegetarians. The average male in India has a cholesterol level of 202 mg, and the average female has a cholesterol level of 208 mg, yet Indo-Asians have the highest rates of heart disease on the planet, and are between 50 and 300 percent more likely to develop heart disease than are Europeans, Americans, and other Asians.

Many studies of statin (cholesterol-lowering) drugs have shown that statins do indeed decrease the risk of another heart attack in heart patients, but the same number of patients end up dying whether they are taking statin drugs or not. A 2006 study in the *Archives of Internal Medicine* reviewed seven trials of statin drugs in nearly forty-three thousand middle-aged men without heart disease. The review showed that taking statins did not lower these patients' mortality levels at all. Dr. Beatrice Golomb, an associate professor of medicine at the University of California, San Francisco, commented on this phenomenon: "You may have helped the heart, but you haven't helped the patient. You still have to look at the impact on the patient overall."

Dr. Mark Ebell, a professor at the University of Georgia, said of statin drugs: "High-risk groups have a lot to gain. But patients at low risk benefit very little if at all. We end up overtreating a lot of patients."

Numerous large-scale studies of people with high cholesterol have shown that when their cholesterol levels are lowered, patients are less likely to die of heart attacks, but more likely to die in traffic accidents, to be murdered, or to commit suicide. Researcher Dr. Vivian Mitropoulu remarked, "A lot of them seemed to be smashing their cars into bridges and doing all sorts of violent and impulsive things." In the end, the patients' odds of dying turned out to be the same whether or not they took cholesterol-lowering drugs.

Other studies have shown that people with extremely low cholesterol levels have higher mortality rates than do people with normal cholesterol levels. One report published in the *Archives of Internal Medicine* in 1992 studied 350,000 healthy middle-aged men; 6 percent of the men in the study had very low cholesterol levels (under 160). According to Dr. James Neaton of the University of Minnesota, the very-low-cholesterol men showed hardly a trace of heart disease during the twelve years of the study, and their death rate from heart attacks was only half that of men who had cholesterol levels of 200 to 239. But these very-low-cholesterol subjects were twice as likely to have bleeding strokes, three times as likely to have liver cancer, twice as likely to die of lung disease, twice as likely to kill themselves, and five times as likely to die of alcoholism as were the men with higher cholesterol levels. Studies in other countries have also shown that very low cholesterol levels increase the risk of death for both men and women.

The relationship between low cholesterol and aggression has even been demonstrated in other species. In 1991, J. R. Kaplan, S. B. Manuck, and C. Shively, of the Department of Comparative Medicine at the Bowman Gray School of Medicine in Winston-Salem, North Carolina, studied the behavior of thirty adult monkeys who were fed either a high-fat, high-cholesterol "luxury" diet, or a low-fat, low-cholesterol "prudent" diet. The high-living monkeys had higher cholesterol levels than did the prudent monkeys. But the prudent monkeys were more aggressive than the high-living monkeys. The researchers concluded: "These results are consistent with studies linking relatively low serum cholesterol concentrations to violent or antisocial behavior in psychiatric and criminal populations and could be relevant to understanding the significant increase in violence-related mortality observed among people assigned to cholesterol-lowering treatment in clinical trials."

## ALL BOTTLED UP

Reports of odd reactions to statin drugs inspired Drs. B. A. Golomb, T. Kane, and J. E. Dimsdale of the University of California, San Diego, to study the psychological effects of statin drugs. They questioned six patients who had reported severe irritability while on statins. Patient One was a sixty-three-year-old male who tried taking statins five different times, but quit each time because of extreme irritability. His chief complaint was "I wanted to kill someone." On several occasions he awoke in a rage, with "uncontrollable pent-up tension" and wanting "to kill someone" and "smash things." He damaged property and stated that he believed that if he had been married, he would have become a widower. When he stopped taking the statin drug, his rage disappeared within two days, and he reverted to his naturally even-tempered and mild personality.

Patient number two tried six different statin drugs over a period of three years. He discontinued the drugs rather rapidly each time because of intolerable "crabbiness" that on two different occasions almost induced him to murder his wife.

One patient had such severe episodes of road rage that he had to stop driving, though he still raged at other drivers from the passenger seat. After three years of anger, he finally stopped taking the statins, and within two weeks recovered his normally placid temperament.

## LOW AND BLUE

Psychologist Edward Suarez of the Duke University Medical Center in Durham, North Carolina, administered psychological tests to 121 healthy women between the ages of eighteen and twenty-seven and found that those with serum cholesterol levels below 160 mg/dl were more likely to develop anxiety and depression than were women who had normal or higher than normal cholesterol levels. (A normal cholesterol level is considered to be between 180 and 200 mg/dl.)

Many previous studies of male subjects had already shown a connection between low cholesterol levels and aggression and depression. (This does not mean that the average person who has fairly low cholesterol levels should go out and gorge himself on butter and bacon—unless he starts feeling murderous, in which case it might be a good idea.)

Taking statin drugs reduces the odds of having a heart attack by 25 percent. But 25 percent of what? If you want help in making an informed decision, go to www.nhlbi.nih.gov/guidelines/cholesterol and use the ten-year risk calculator, which will estimate your odds of having a heart attack. If your chances are fifty-fifty, taking statin drugs might seem like a good option. On the other hand, if your risk is already low, a 25 percent reduction may be almost meaningless.

## DRUG$

The statin drugs are very, very heavily advertised not because the pharmaceutical companies are concerned about your health and well-being, but because the companies are interested in their own bottom line. And statins have been wonderful for their bottom line. In 2002, pharmaceutical companies sold $12.5 billion worth of statin drugs in the United States alone. Even at the lowest dosages, Pfizer's Lipitor, the best-selling statin drug, costs more than a dollar per pill. In fact, Lipitor is so lucrative that between 2006 and 2008, Pfizer was able to spend more than $258 million on an advertising campaign that featured Dr. Robert Jarvik, who was billed as the inventor of the artificial heart. Pfizer's patent for Lipitor expires in 2010, and the company apparently wanted to strengthen consumer loyalty for the brand name before the generic versions of the drug hit the market.

The ads featured Dr. Jarvik introducing himself, talking about his invention, the artificial heart, and recommending Lipitor. One ad showed him running with his son, and another showed him rowing a racing shell expertly across a mountain lake. Everything went swimmingly until the advertising campaign was called into question by a congressional committee examining drug advertising aimed at consumers. During the hearings it was revealed that though Jarvik is a medical doctor, he is not a cardiologist and he has never practiced medicine on actual patients.

Several of Jarvik's colleagues challenged his assertion that he invented the artificial heart, and stated that the original "Jarvik heart" was a modified version of a colleague's prototype. Apparently Jarvik does not row, so for advertising purposes a body double had impersonated the doctor rowing across the mountain lake. After the congressional hearings, Pfizer withdrew the Lipitor ads that featured Dr. Jarvik. Beware drug companies bearing big advertising budgets.

## CHOLESTEROL ON MY MIND

Cholesterol has been blamed for almost all heart disease for nearly a century. But where did this idea come from? Is cholesterol really completely bad?

In 1909, Dr. A. Ignatowski investigated the effects of a high-protein, high-fat, high-cholesterol diet on laboratory rabbits. Dr. Ignatowski fed his rabbits large amounts of meat, eggs, and milk. The diet damaged the livers and adrenal glands (which are associated with the kidneys) of young rabbits. The diet caused older rabbits to develop arterial lesions that looked remarkably like atherosclerosis in humans. Later researchers enlarged and elaborated upon the cholesterol-causes-heart-disease theory.

I am fairly sure that I, an omnivorous primate, would fare badly on the tree bark diet that our local rabbits subsist on in the winter, and I am not at all surprised that herbivores such as rabbits do not thrive on a carnivorous diet.

### BEWARE THE DEADLY SEVENTH EGG

In April 2008, researchers Dr. Luc Djousse and Dr. J. Michael Gaziano, of Brigham and Women's Hospital and Harvard Medical School, reported the results of their study of the eating habits and mortality rates of 21,327 male physicians who were participating in the Physicians' Health Study. The researchers found that "Whereas egg consumption of up to six eggs a week was not associated with the risk of all-cause mortality, consumption of (seven or more) eggs a week was associated with a 23 percent greater risk of death."

Dr. Robert Eckel, former president of the American Heart Association, commented: "It's really hard to say at this point, but it still seems, if you're a middle-aged male physician and enjoy eggs more than once a day, that having some of the egg left on your face may be better than having it go down your gullet."

However, Dr. Djousse and Dr. Gaziano did notice that the men who ate seven or more eggs per week were also older, fatter, more likely to drink alcohol, more likely to smoke, and less likely to exercise than were the men who ate fewer eggs.

Apparently, the moral of the story is that if you plan to grow older, fatter, and lazier while continuing to smoke, drink, and overeat, you should limit your egg intake to six per week.

Despite nearly unrelenting bad publicity, cholesterol is here to stay, because we humans, like all other vertebrates, simply cannot live without it.

The membranes that surround all our cells are rich in cholesterol, which helps keep the membranes in good condition. Cholesterol-rich membranes are flexible, fluid, and permeable, so that nutrients can easily enter the cell and waste products can readily exit it. A cell membrane that is low in cholesterol may partially solidify and become less permeable.

Cholesterol is one of the main components of the myelin sheathing that insulates our nerve cells, allowing impulses to travel quickly, smoothly, and efficiently along the nerve bundles. One quarter of all the cholesterol in our bodies is in our brains, mostly in the sheathing around the nerve cells. In fact, if you dry out a human brain and then weigh it, cholesterol will make up about half its dry weight.

Cholesterol is the raw material that our bodies use to synthesize the following substances:

Vitamin D, which regulates calcium and phosphorus metabolism. When sunshine hits our skin it converts cholesterol to vitamin D.

Steroid hormones that help us metabolize sugars, cope with stress, and regulate our blood pressure.

The sex hormones, which make us either masculine or feminine and allow us to reproduce.

Even the humble bile salts that allow us to digest fats are made from cholesterol.

Only 25 percent of our serum cholesterol comes from our food; we synthesize the remaining 75 percent in our livers.

Statin drugs lower serum cholesterol levels by interfering with the liver's ability to synthesize cholesterol.

More and more researchers are coming to the conclusion that inflammation can make the plaques on artery walls break loose. These unfettered plaques may induce the formation of blood clots that can cause strokes and heart attacks. But what causes all this inflammation? In 400 B.C., the Greek physician Hippocrates observed, "Sudden death is more common in those who are naturally fat than in the lean." Many modern researchers who have studied the relationship between obesity and cardiovascular disease have come to the conclusion that excess avoirdupois, especially in the midsection, induces systemic inflammation. Clinical weight loss studies have shown that as people lose body fat, their levels of inflammation drop.

Two-thirds of Americans are already overweight, and the incidence of obesity is rapidly increasing. The number of Americans who are afflicted with heart disease, high blood pressure, diabetes, and other weight-related disorders is expected to swell to fifty million in the next several years as the number of obese Americans balloons. In March 2008, Consumers Union estimated that approximately twenty million Americans are already taking statin drugs to lower their cholesterol levels. If you are quiet, and listen intently, you may be able to hear the pharmaceutical industry rubbing its sticky hands together in gleeful anticipation of ballooning profits.

## CHRONIC PAIN

When I tore my anterior cruciate ligament (ACL) about ten years ago, the emergency room doctors told me not to put any weight on it, and to go see my own doctor in a week. Unfortunately, I did as they said. By the time I visited my doctor a week later, the skin of my affected leg had gotten so exquisitely tender that the slightest touch had become excruciating. I couldn't bear the bedsheet touching my leg, and you could literally have knocked me down by brushing my leg with a feather. My doctor sent me to a surgeon, who told me that I could put full weight on my knee while I waited for surgery. As soon as I started using my leg again, the skin pain disappeared. I imagine that the scenario might have gone something like this:

Worried by the absence of a normal amount of feedback from the leg, the brain turns the volume way up on the nerves in the leg: "Brain to Leg. Brain to Leg. Come in, Leg. Are you there?" Nothing. Brain turns up the volume on the body radio and tries again: "Brain to Leg. Brain to Leg. Come in, Leg." Nothing. Brain turns up the volume again, and then Leg brushes up against the bedsheet, which causes an excruciating feedback loop. "*Aaaaah!*"

So when I began reading about complex regional pain syndrome (CRPS), it sounded a bit familiar. CRPS can cause skin hypersensitivity, asymmetrical temperature and color changes in the skin, swelling and sweating, burning and stinging pain, stiffness, tremors, and weakness. CRPS can even cause changes in the way the skin, fingernails, and hair grow. Fabric lightly brushing against the skin, wind blowing across the skin, and even moderately cool or warm temperatures can cause pain.

CRPS often starts after a person has been injured. The injury causes pain, the patient restricts her movements in order to avoid the pain, and often, just as full recovery seems near, excruciating pain sets in and stays. Therapists have learned that normal movement is vital in the recovery of CRPS patients. Though pain is usually an important signal that something is wrong, CRPS pain is just pain; there is no underlying organic problem— the alarm is still going off after the fire has been extinguished.

Researchers in Scotland and Sweden have found that brushing the skin reduced the excitability of the muscles under the skin. They hope that this phenomenon can be used in the treatment of pain.

I wish I had known about skin brushing ten years ago!

Phantom pain is pain that is felt in a missing limb, and can be severe and disabling. At least 90 percent of limb amputees have phantom limb pain, and two-thirds of amputees still experience phantom pain eight years after they have lost a limb. Up to 70 percent of phantom limbs remain painful after twenty-five years. Scientists believe that the pain is caused by brain reorganization (remapping) that occurs after the amputation. This remapping confuses the brain into thinking it is getting feedback from a limb that is no longer there. When the limb is quite obviously not behaving normally, the brain activates the pain signals.

In 1994, Dr. Vilayanus S. Ramachandran, a professor of neuroscience at the University of California–San Diego, devised a treatment for a twenty-eight-year-old man who had lost his left arm in a motorcycle accident ten years previously. The phantom arm felt paralyzed, pressed into the patient's body, and it had ached horribly for ten years. Dr. Ramachandran built a simple device consisting of a box that was open at the top and the front, with a vertical mirror mounted in the middle. The patient put his right arm in the box, and the mirror gave the illusion that his missing left arm was also in the box. Dr. Ramachandran asked the patient to make symmetrical movements with both hands, as if he were conducting an orchestra, and the patient yelled: "Oh, my God, my wrist is moving, my elbow is moving." When asked to close his eyes, the phantom limb felt paralyzed once again. Dr. Ramachandran sent the patient home with the box and told him to play around with it.

Three weeks later, Dr. Ramachandran received a phone call, which he recounted like this:

> "Doctor, it's gone!
> "What's gone"
> "My phantom arm is gone."
> "What?"
> "All I have is fingers and a lower palm dangling from my shoulder."
> "Does this bother you?"
> "No. The pain in my elbow is gone. I can move my fingers. But your box doesn't work anymore."

Since then, doctors have used mirrors to rid other sufferers of phantom limb pain, and lately the technique has become more high tech as researchers utilize virtual reality systems to give patients the illusion that their missing limb is functioning normally.

The latest hypothesis is that mirror therapy and virtual reality therapy work due to the activation of mirror neurons in the brain. These neurons fire either when a person performs an action or when he observes another person performing an action. When the phantom limb appears to be operating normally the "All's well" message suppresses the pain pathways, and the brain begins to rewire itself so that the pain, and sometimes the phantom limb itself, is reduced or disappears entirely.

Researchers are now studying whether virtual reality systems can also be used to treat other disorders that are caused by miscommunication between the sensory and motor systems, such as fibromyalgia, myofascitis, chronic pain syndromes, and headache.

Once the brain has been convinced that all is well with the body, it begins to rewire itself and eventually eliminates the persistent pain.

## A REAL PAIN IN THE BACK

Herta Flor, Ph.D., of the University of Heidelberg in Germany, used electroencephalograms (EEGs) to track the way chronic pain sufferers respond to pain. The 2002 study, however, had an unusual twist. The researchers recruited chronic pain sufferers as well as their spouses: ten chronic pain sufferers with their solicitous spouses; ten chronic pain sufferers whose spouses were not solicitous; and ten healthy subjects who did not suffer from back pain. The solicitous spouses had a history of being very attentive to their suffering partners' pain. The nonsolicitous spouses did not dwell on their partners' pain, and tended to try to distract them and keep them from thinking about it.

When the researchers administered painful electric shocks to the backs of chronic pain sufferers, the presence of solicitous spouses made the back pain worse—two and a half times worse! When the solicitous spouses were not in the room, the intensity of their mates' pain decreased. The presence of non-solicitous spouses did not increase the intensity of their spouses' back pain.

According to Flor, "The findings show that the solicitous spouse has become a cue for a more intense pain experience in the back." Apparently, pain feeds on attention.

## THE DOCTOR'S MICROSCOPIC HELPERS

"The microbial part of ourselves is highly evolved. These organisms
have learned to adapt to life with us."
—Jeffrey Gordon, microbiologist, Washington University,
St. Louis, Missouri

Though every human being begins life as a germ-free fetus floating in his mother's sea, he picks up millions of bacteria as he exits her body. A normal, healthy human is a symbiont whose human cells are outnumbered ten to one by microbial cells, and whose health is completely interwoven with and dependent upon its microbial community.

Researchers at the National Human Genome Research Institute reckon that there are at least twenty distinct ecological niches for microbes on the skin surface of the average human being. The microbial community of the inner elbow is entirely different from that of the inner forearm, only inches away. The microbes that live on the front of the teeth differ from those that live on the dark side, and different species of bacteria may live in the gum pockets around two adjacent teeth.

Some microbial communities are more helpful than others. Dr. Johannes Aas, Dr. Charles E. Gessert, and Dr. Johan S. Bakken of St. Mary's Clinic in Duluth, Minnesota, have been using a novel method to cure patients who are suffering from recurrent attacks of infectious colitis. Their patients were infected by Clostridium difficile, which are very dangerous, frequently antibiotic-resistant bacteria that are capable of destroying the colon if left untreated.

This is the treatment: The doctors collect a stool sample from a healthy donor (preferably the patient's spouse), plop it into a blender along with sterile salt water, and blend until smooth. They filter the suspension through a paper coffee filter and then filter it again. The resulting liquid is administered to the patient via a nasogastric tube. This inoculation of normal bacteria helps restore the patients' colonic ecosystem to health. The doctors have had a success rate of between 94 and 100 percent with their low-tech fecal bacteriotherapy method. Other researchers use the enema method to administer the beneficial liquid.

Though it is aesthetically unappealing, fecal bacteriotherapy is becoming fairly common worldwide; it is the most reliable treatment yet devised for patients who have been infected by Clostridium difficile.

## GET DIRTY, BE HAPPY

Mycobacterium vaccae, a harmless bacteria normally found in dirt, has been successfully deployed as a vaccine against tuberculosis, and is being tested as a treatment for cancer, asthma, allergies, and as a way to reboot the immune system.

Cancer researcher Mary O'Brian, of the Royal Marsden Hospital in London, England, was testing M. vaccae as a treatment for human lung cancer. Cancer patients were inoculated with heat-killed preparations of the bacteria. The bacterial treatment helped reduce the patients' cancer symptoms, but the researchers were quite surprised when they noticed that their patients were also livelier, happier, and more mentally acute.

Christopher Lowry, a neuroscientist at the University of Bristol, U.K., was intrigued by O'Brian's study, and decided to study how M. vaccae affects the brain. Lowry and his colleagues injected heat-killed M. *vac-cae* into a group of mice and found that the bacteria initiated an immune response that activated serotonin-producing neurons in the brain. Low levels of serotonin cause depression. In 2007, Lowry noted that the studies "leave us wondering if we shouldn't all spend more time playing in the dirt."

## THE DOCTOR'S LITTLE HELPERS

The practice of using living animals or microorganisms to treat or diagnose disease is now called biotherapy. It used to be called practicing medicine. It is believed that leeches were first used medicinally as early as 1500 B.C. In fact, doctors used to be referred to as "leeches" because they so frequently used leeches on their patients.

Leeches were used very commonly in the nineteenth century A.D. for bloodletting, which was believed to be a cure for everything from headaches to gout. As medical science advanced, doctors used medicinal leeches less and less frequently, and the practice of leeching was commonly regarded as quaint, old-fashioned, and possibly dangerous. Then in 1960, two Slovenian surgeons, M. Derganc and F. Zdravic, published a paper in the *British Journal of Plastic Surgery* in which they described using leeches to maintain the circulation and prevent gangrene after skin graft surgery.

Since the publication of that groundbreaking paper, the use of medicinal leeches has been steadily increasing. Recent studies have shown that transplanted flaps of skin tissue are much more likely to thrive when treated with leeches than they are when treated with drugs or with surgery alone.

In June 2004, the Food and Drug Administration officially approved leeches for use as medical devices. The FDA's definition of a medical device is "an article intended to diagnose, cure, treat, prevent, or mitigate a disease or condition, or to affect a function or structure of the body, that does not achieve its primary effect through a chemical action and is not metabolized."

Leech saliva contains substances that anesthetize the wound area, dilate the blood vessels, increase blood flow, and prevent blood from clotting and pooling in the injured area. All of these properties are quite useful when a surgeon is battling to reattach and save a severed appendage. Nearly miraculous reattachment surgeries of fingers, hands, toes, legs, ears, noses, and scalps have been accomplished with the postoperative help of leeches. Leeches have also been used to treat less dramatic injuries such as black eyes and hematomas (masses of clotted blood). Unlike common pond or swamp leeches, medicinal leeches are raised at special farms under tightly controlled, disease-free conditions. After they do their job, the engorged medicinal leeches are discarded along with the infectious waste.

Disgust is an emotion that most of us cannot afford to indulge in while dealing with an emergency. Hand surgery specialist Dr. Vincent Hentz of Stanford University said of his professional leech experiences: "Patients have a lot invested in a thumb or a hand. There's never been a patient who's declined. Most are enthusiastic, and some start naming their leeches."

## MAGGOTS

During the American Civil War, field surgeons noticed that soldiers whose wounds were crawling with blowfly maggots were less likely to develop gangrene and more likely to survive than were their fellows whose wounds were not infested with maggots. A Confederate army surgeon named J. F. Zacharias began using maggots to clean out soldiers' wounds. He wrote: "Maggots, in a single day, would clean a wound much better than any agents we had at our command. I am sure I saved many lives by their use."

During the First World War, military surgeons observed that injured soldiers who reached the field hospital several days after being wounded on far-off battlefields had a better survival rate if they had maggots in their wounds. During the war, Dr. William S. Baer, an orthopedic consultant to the American forces in France, treated two soldiers who had been left lying wounded on a battlefield for a week after the battle ended. Baer was astonished that their maggot-infested compound fractures and abdominal wounds had already begun to heal and showed no signs of infection. Ten years later, at Johns Hopkins University, Professor Baer became one of the first modern practitioners of maggot therapy when he began treating chronic skin and bone infections by introducing maggots into the open wounds.

In the 1940s, with the advent of antibiotics, maggots fell out of fashion. Maggot therapy was occasionally used during the 1970s and 1980s, but only when antibiotics, surgery, and high-tech wound care had failed to control an infection. Now that we are entering the postantibiotic era, maggots are back in style. The first modern clinical studies of maggot therapy were begun in 1989 at the Veterans Affairs Medical Center in Long Beach, California. The results were so encouraging that physicians there have been using maggot therapy earlier, rather than waiting until all other options have failed.

But don't try this at home! Only a few species of maggots, primarily larvae of blowflies, are suitable for maggot therapy duty—these maggots prefer decomposing tissue; they avoid the live, healthy stuff. The maggots dissolve and remove dead tissue, and then eat the liquefied tissue, and bacteria—even the nastiest, antibiotic-resistant varieties of bacteria—cannot survive the onslaught.

Wounds that are commonly treated with maggot therapy include leg and foot ulcers, chronic diabetic ulcers, pressure sores, burns, and postoperative wounds that have reopened after becoming infected. One woman, who had a gangrenous perforated bowel, was successfully treated with the help of thousands of eager maggots. The maggots obliterated all traces of gangrene and the patient made a complete recovery.

## A FISHY STORY

In the 1960s, some of the people who frequented the therapeutic hot springs in Kangal, Turkey, reported that small, toothless fish had nibbled away at and removed their calluses, hardened skin, and even the hard, thick, scaly plaques caused by psoriasis (an inflammatory skin disorder). The heat-tolerant "doctor fish" are members of two different species in the carp family, *Cyprinion macrostomus* and *Garra rufa obtusa,* and are known as "Strikers" and "Lickers," respectively.

The little fish wait until the hot water has softened the bathers up a little, then attack and eat their dead and/or damaged skin. The doctor fish are reportedly very good for helping relieve the discomfort of psoriasis.

More recently, spas around the world have begun importing doctor fish and are offering "fish pedicures" and "fish massages" to their callused clients.

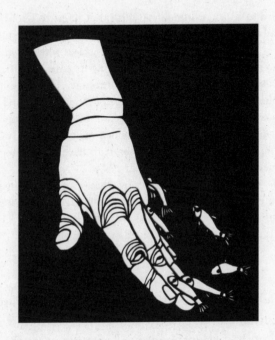

## WORM-RIDDEN

Over the past half century, a precipitous rise in the incidence of inflammatory bowel disease (IBD) in wealthy countries has coincided with a precipitous plunge in the number of citizens whose guts are inhabited by parasites such as roundworms, pinworms, and human whipworms. In developing countries, these parasites are nearly ubiquitous, and IBD, Crohn's disease, and ulcerative colitis are rare.

In the 1990s, Dr. Joel Weinstock, director of the Digestive Disease Center at the University of Iowa Hospitals and Clinics, in Iowa City, observed the coincidence between the rise of autoimmune bowel diseases and the fall of intestinal parasites, and decided to do something about it. Dr. Weinstock believed that the immune system becomes hyperactive when it has no parasites to fight, so he devised a small study in which volunteers who were suffering from IBD drank Gatorade that contained the microscopic eggs of porcine whipworms, *Trichuris suis*.

Inflammatory bowel disease is a portmanteau term that refers to Crohn's disease, ulcerative colitis, and other autoimmune disorders that affect the digestive system.

Crohn's disease is an autoimmune disorder that causes inflammation of the digestive tract. It can affect the digestive tract all along its entire length, though it most commonly affects the lower part of the small intestine. The swelling and scar tissue caused by Crohn's disease can form a blockage of the intestine, and the sores, abscesses, and ulcers can perforate the intestine or form fistulas that tunnel through to surrounding areas and cause infections of the bladder, vagina, or skin. Two-thirds to three-quarters of patients with Crohn's disease eventually have part of their intestine removed, and most need surgery more than once.

Ulcerative colitis is an autoimmune disorder that causes inflammation and ulcerations in the lining of the colon and rectum. Between 25 and 40 percent of ulcerative colitis patients must eventually have their colons removed because of massive bleeding, severe illness, rupture of the colon, or risk of cancer.

Dr. Weinstock chose porcine whipworms because they are relatively short-lived creatures that can live in the human digestive tract but cannot reproduce there. All of the patients improved after ingesting the whipworm eggs; most patients went into complete remission, and a few were able to discontinue their drugs. The volunteers had to drink another round of worm eggs every three weeks, or their symptoms returned. After Dr. Weinstock's study was published in 1999, he was deluged with calls from desperate IBD patients who wanted to drink porcine whipworm eggs.

In 2004, Weinstock released the results of a larger study that tested the effects of porcine whipworms on two hundred volunteers, half of whom had Crohn's disease, while the other half had ulcerative colitis. Half the ulcerative colitis patients and 70 percent of the Crohn's patients went into remission after being treated with whipworms.

A German company named BioCure (whose sister company, BioMonde, sells leeches and maggots) found the results so convincing that they dove into the whipworm business. They plan to sell a salutary whipworm cocktail under the name TSO, which stands for *Trichuris Suis* Ova. TSO may be easier to market than PWE (Pig Whipworm Eggs).

About a year ago, while I was giving a vermicomposting talk, a member of the audience expressed her concerns about the possibility of contracting parasitic worms from a vermicomposting bin. She had just returned from a trip to Two Harbors, Minnesota, which was in the throes of a pinworm epidemic, and she was feeling squeamish. I assured her that earthworms and pinworms are not the same type of worm, and that it was unlikely that anyone would acquire pinworms from a worm bin unless a pinworm-infested person had used that worm bin as a latrine. I then talked about the inverse relationship between intestinal worms and inflammatory bowel disease and Crohn's disease. To my horror, three out of the ten people in the room were very close to at least one person who had either died of Crohn's disease or who had undergone multiple surgeries to remove sections of intestine that had been damaged by Crohn's disease. Since then, every time I have mentioned this topic, at least two people reveal that they have loved ones who are suffering from Crohn's disease.

Pinworms are relatively innocuous—they only cause a little bit of hind-end itching. Perhaps Two Harbors should launch an annual Pinworm Festival.

## HOOKED ON HELMINTHS

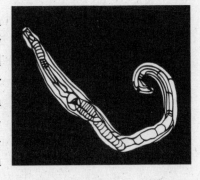

In 2004, Dr. David Pritchard, an immunologist-biologist at the University of Nottingham, U.K., purposefully infected himself with intestinal hookworms in order to test a theory and to obtain permission from the National Health Service to conduct helminth therapy studies on volunteers. (Parasitic intestinal worms are known as helminths.)

While carrying out fieldwork in Papua New Guinea in the late 1980s, Dr. Pritchard had noticed that Papuans who were infected with intestinal hookworms seemed immune to autoimmune disorders such as hay fever and asthma. Dr. Pritchard developed a theory to explain the phenomenon: "The allergic response evolved to help expel parasites, and we think the worms have found a way of switching off the immune system in order to survive. That's why infected people have fewer allergic symptoms."

Dr. Pritchard recruited thirty volunteers, fifteen of whom received ten hookworms apiece. After six weeks, the fifteen worm hosts had begun to produce lower levels of inflammatory chemicals. The worm-bearers were wildly enthusiastic as their allergy symptoms began disappearing. Word soon spread online, and a Yahoo group on "helminthic therapy" was formed. For more information on helminthic therapy and for links to groups, go to www.helminthictherapy.com.

According to Dr. Pritchard: "Many of the people who were given a placebo have requested worms, and many of the people with worms have elected to keep them."

## DIABETIC MICE

Non-obese diabetic (NOD) mice have been used in diabetes research for more than twenty years. A large percentage of these specially bred mice can be relied upon to develop type 1 diabetes, an autoimmune disorder that causes the body's immune system to attack and eventually destroy the beta cells of the pancreas. NOD mice have also demonstrated a remarkable talent for developing a wide range of other autoimmune disorders. In a study published in the June 2007 issue of *Diabetes*, researchers Krishnan Sundar, Qian Liu, Gitty Mousavi, William C. Gause, and David Bleich demonstrated that infecting infant NOD mice with parasitic worms (helminths) helped protect the mice from developing type 1 diabetes. At three months of age, 70 percent of worm-free NOD mice had developed diabetes, while only 10 percent of their worm-infested fellows had developed diabetes.

The researchers concluded that helminth infection regulated the immune response of the mice and diverted the immune cells' destructive attention away from the beta cells of the pancreas.

## NETTLED

The ancient Romans considered a good flogging with stinging nettles (*Urtica dioica* and *Urtica urens*) to be a cure for chronic rheumatism. The treatment was called urtication. In the year A.D. 2000, scientists took nettles out for a test flog and liked what they saw.

Researchers from the University of Plymouth, Devon, U.K., conducted a randomized controlled study on twenty-seven patients who had osteo-arthritic pain at the base of the thumb or index finger. The volunteers rubbed their hands either with stinging nettle leaf (*Urtica dioica*), or with the leaves of the look-alike white dead nettle (*Lamium album*). Eventually, over the course of the ten-week study, all the volunteers experienced the effects of both types of leaves. All the volunteers were told that they were helping to investigate the effects of two different types of nettle, and that they might feel some slight but harmless stinging. The stinging nettles gave the arthritis sufferers significant pain relief; the dead nettle treatment had no effect.

Fourteen of the twenty-seven patients preferred the stinging nettle treatment to their usual analgesics, and seventeen wanted to use the treatment in the future.

The researchers noted that the stiff, stinging hairs of the stinging nettle contain serotonin, acetylcholine, histamine, and leukotrienes.

My friend Lynda was a professional dancer until she ruined her knees. She has had multiple knee surgeries and is often in pain. I urticated her knees one fine summer day several years ago, and she was pleased with the results. The nettles raised some welts, but made her knee joints feel better.

## DISGUSTINGLY HEALTHY

It is interesting to note that when people are truly suffering, their squea-mishness flies right out the window. Suddenly, phenomena that would have been the stuff of their worst nightmares becomes the subject of their fondest dreams. When faced with the choice of losing a limb to gangrene, or letting maggots chew on that limb, everyone chooses the maggots. Excruciating intestinal pain or intestinal worms? Everyone wants worms.

Green Barbarians know that insulating themselves from the natural world is a prescription for disaster, and they live and act accordingly.

## Chapter Seven

# Barbarian Pets

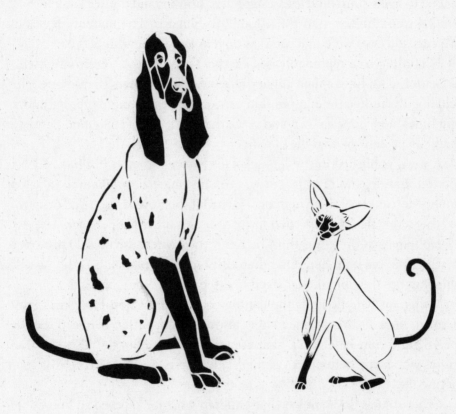

## OF CANARIES, CANINES, AND CATS

You may have more in common with your pet than you think. A 1991 study conducted by the National Research Council determined that illness in pets can be a sign that there is something wrong with their home environment, and their owners are also at risk.

In 2008, the Environmental Working Group tested blood and urine samples from thirty-five dogs and thirty-seven cats. The results were rather alarming.

## DOGS

The dogs were contaminated with thirty-five different chemicals, including eleven carcinogens, thirty-one reproductive toxins, and twenty-four neurotoxins. The canine levels of perfluorochemicals (the toxic chemicals that are used to make stain- and grease-repellent finishes and nonstick cookware) were 2.4 times higher than those found in humans. The mercury levels in both cats and dogs were five times as high as those found in people.

According to a report released by the Texas A&M Veterinary Medical Center, dogs have much higher rates of many cancers than do people, including thirty-five times more skin cancer, four times more breast tumors, eight times more bone cancer, and twice the incidence of leukemia. Between 20 and 25 percent of dogs die of cancer.

A study published in the *Journal of the National Cancer Institute* in 1991 reported that dogs were at least two or more times more likely to develop lymphoma (cancer of the lymphatic system) if their owners sprayed or sprinkled the herbicide 2,4-D on their lawns four or more times per year. The risk of lymphoma was only one-third higher if the owners used 2,4-D just once per season. (This is an herbicide that kills broadleaf plants; it is the "weed" component of the ubiquitous "weed-and-feed" lawn care products.)

Malignant lymphoma is the canine equivalent of non-Hodgkin's lymphoma in humans. Many researchers suspect a connection between the use of 2,4-D and non-Hodgkin's lymphoma; several studies have shown that farmers who spray herbicides on their fields have an increased risk of contracting the disease.

Other studies have shown that children who are exposed to household pesticides and lawn and garden chemicals at home also have a greatly increased risk of developing non-Hodgkin's lymphoma, childhood leukemia, brain cancer, neuroblastoma, Wilms' tumor, soft-tissue sarcoma, Ewing's sarcoma, and cancers of the brain, colorectum, and testes. According to a 1998 study conducted by Sheila Hoar Zahm and Mary H. Ward of the National Cancer Institute in Rockville, Maryland, household chemicals pose a much greater risk to children than they do to adults. Children's small size, fast growth rates, rapid respiration, and high metabolic rates mean that they absorb more toxins per unit of body weight than adults do, and children's immature immune systems are ill equipped to deal effectively with many of the toxins they absorb. Zahm and Ward concluded: "There is potential to prevent at least some childhood cancer by reducing or eliminating pesticide exposure."

Apparently the word is not getting out. Over the last decade, I have had many people tell me that their neighbors next door, across the street, or around the corner just brought their child home from the hospital where he or she had been treated for leukemia. They told their neighbors that there is a connection between childhood leukemia and lawn chemicals, so they might want to cancel their lawn service. Their neighbors are still using the lawn service. The first time I was told this story, I was shocked and dismayed. The second time, I was a little less surprised. Now I am simply disgusted. I am not hearing about the same family over and over—apparently there is an epidemic of Americans who love their lawns more than they love their children.

On the other hand, pet owners sometimes get the message. I have had a few people tell me that after years of trying, they were finally able to persuade their parents to stop using lawn chemicals, but only after their parents' dogs had died of cancer. One of the canine victims had actually developed cancer in the pads of her paws!

## CATS

The feline blood donors for the Environmental Working Group's chemical study were contaminated with forty-six chemicals, including nine carcinogens, forty reproductive toxins, thirty-four neurotoxins, and fifteen endocrine toxins. Polybrominated diphenyl ethers (PBDEs), which are suspected endocrine toxins that are used as flame retardants, were found in concentrations that were twenty-three times as high as those commonly found in humans.

Feline hypothyroidism is a frequently fatal disease that was relatively rare until the 1980s, when it suddenly became much more common. Feline hypothyroidism is now a leading cause of cat death.

In the 1980s, manufacturers began using large volumes of brominated flame retardants in consumer products such as mattresses, furniture cushions, carpet padding, and electronics. PBDEs mimic thyroid hormones, so many experts suspect that high exposure to PBDEs can overstimulate cats' thyroids. PBDE levels have been increasing in the environment, in people, and in wildlife for the past two decades, especially in the United States, where levels are the highest in the world, and have been doubling every few years.

In 2007, EPA researchers tested blood samples from twenty-three cats, including eleven with hyperthyroidism. Although all of the cats had PBDEs in their blood, the cats with thyroid disease had higher average PBDE concentrations.

Though canned seafood and fish-flavored catfood may contain high levels of PBDEs, much of the contamination in felines and in humans enters our bodies in the form of dust. Cats often come into direct and prolonged contact with upholstery, carpeting, and mattresses that contain flame retardants, and often sit on electronic equipment. The researchers noted in their report that because of their meticulous grooming behavior, cats may ingest large amounts of dust, and added that toddlers who crawl on floors and put objects in their mouths could also have very high exposure to chemical-laden dust, which has been found in most American homes.

Two pervasive PBDEs, which were mostly used to flameproof foam cushions, mattresses, and carpet padding, have been banned in the United States since 2004, but other brominated flame retardants are still in widespread use.

As polyurethane foam ages, it begins to break down and turn to dust. Unlike wood-based furniture components, such as plywood and particleboard, which gradually mellow and become less toxic, petroleum-based foam products become more dangerous as they age. Foam made of real latex rubber, and cushion- and mattress-stuffings made of natural materials such as horsehair, wool, cotton, and excelsior, are nontoxic alternatives to toxic cushion- and mattress-stuffings, and are inherently less flammable than cushions made of spongy, solidified gasoline. If we choose safer furnishings, our cats are probably not the only ones whose health will improve. (Cotton-stuffed futons are the safest inexpensive choice for sleepy Green Barbarians on a budget. All the other natural stuffing materials are quite expensive. And it is easy to tell if a used futon is stuffed with cotton: Cotton never springs back on its own, and a used cotton futon is likely to be drastically flattened in its weight-bearing areas.)

## CANARY IN A COAL MINE

Canaries were once used as living air-quality monitors in mines, because the tiny, feathered creatures succumbed quickly when the air became contaminated by toxic fumes. When the canary tumbled off its perch, it was time to evacuate the mine.

Bird owners are often the first people to notice the hazards of various modern materials, and were among the first to raise the alarm about the toxicity of nonstick pots and pans. If you are concerned about the toxicity of a specific material, try visiting the website www.birdsandmore.com and check to see whether there are any reports that the product has killed pet birds. Any product that emits a strong chemical odor may endanger an indoor bird. If your air quality is good enough to keep a caged bird healthy, it's probably good enough for you, too.

Among the products that have killed pet birds are insecticidal foggers and household sprays; hair sprays, perfumes, air fresheners, and overheated nonstick pans; automobile exhaust; tobacco smoke; glue and paint fumes; air fresheners; scented candles and "long-burning" candles, which often have wicks that have been stiffened with lead wire. (EPA tests have shown that candles with lead wicks can raise the level of lead in the air to a concentration that is high enough to cause instantaneous death in birds.)

## LAWN BIRDS

According to the National Audubon Society and the U.S. Fish and Wildlife Service, lawn chemicals kill approximately seven million birds annually in the United States. Direct exposure to pesticides on farm fields kills an estimated sixty-seven million birds annually, and millions more die when they eat poisoned bugs or small animals.

Many cases of avian pesticide poisoning go unreported, because the victims stagger off to die hidden and alone, or their bodies are squashed by cars, eaten by scavengers (who may then die of pesticide poisoning), or are obliterated by insects and decay; even the carcasses that are noticed are not necessarily sent to a lab for analysis because the tiny victims are found on individual lawns. But when large numbers of big birds drop in a small area, people tend to notice. For instance, in 1972, 500 widgeon ducks died at Seal Beach, California—toxic levels of the pesticide diazinon were detected in the victims' gizzards and in the golf course turf. In 1976, approximately 100 assorted widgeons and coots died of diazinon poisoning at a golf course in Los Alamitos, California, one month after the golf course had been treated with diazinon. And in 1984, up to 40 widgeons died of diazinon poisoning on a different golf course in Southern California. But finally, in 1988, more than 700 Atlantic Brant geese landed on a golf course at Seawane Harbor Golf Course on Long Island, New York, shortly after several of the fairways had been treated with diazinon. That evening, approximately 300 geese were found dead on the fairways and in the nearby harbor. During the next few days a total of 546 dead geese were collected on land, and more birds died in the harbor. An estimated 700 birds died in the incident. Apparently the geese were too big to ignore, because shortly thereafter the EPA banned the use of diazinon on golf courses. Twelve years later the agency finally banned all use of diazinon in the United States.

But I wouldn't plan to roll in the grass on the fairways just yet; pesticides and 2,4-D and other herbicides are still legal and are still sold over the counter. In her book *101 Ways to Help Birds*, bird maven Laura Erickson wrote about an encounter with a homeowner who brought her two violently ill baby robins: "One was on its side, unable to balance itself. Neither could lift its head to beg for food. Both of them trembled with violent spasms every few minutes." The woman told Ms. Erickson that she had found one adult robin dead beneath the nest and another adult and two babies dead inside the nest. When asked whether any lawns had been recently sprayed in the vicinity, the homeowner replied: "Why yes! We sprayed our yard just yesterday. But it can't be that—those chemicals were approved by the EPA." The lawn had been sprayed with "weed-and-feed," and the parent birds must have harvested worms from the poisoned ground and then brought the contaminated harvest home. Both the young birds were dead within a few hours.

If a product is designed to kill, one should usually assume that it's poisonous. We are all earthlings; if a chemical poison will kill a dandelion, crabgrass, fungus, an ant, a cockroach, or a grub, it's probably not good for you or your loved ones either.

## PRIORITIES

If you can't decide whether a lush, green lawn or a healthy pet is more important to you, you need a stuffed animal, not a live pet.

CHAPTER EIGHT

# Little Barbarians

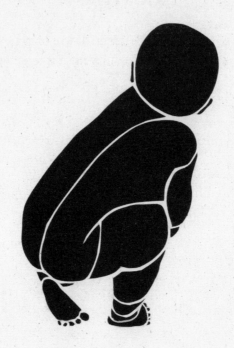

## SQUEAMISHNESS

If you are finicky, particular, or squeamish, you probably shouldn't have children, at least not children who are your direct blood descendants, since the entire reproductive process from beginning to end can be quite sloppy and gooey. If you do decide to adopt, you might want to wait until those children reach the age of reason (thirty-five or so) before you welcome them into your family, because infants, babies, and children are messy, extremely messy.

In case you haven't spent any time around infants, babies, or small children lately, here is the rundown. A very young infant generally needs to have its entire wardrobe changed at least two dozen times every day because it has thoroughly besmirched itself with urine, poop, snot, spit-up milk, tears, and sometimes all of the above simultaneously. Three seconds after you have bathed and dried the infant, it will be sticky again, because infants exude baby glue from all their folds and creases. Older children also secrete many novel substances, some of which they will actively and gleefully share with you. My children were still wiping their noses on me when they were in junior high school.

Infants, babies, and very young children do not, in fact, feel pain in the same way older humans do; their nervous systems are immature and not yet efficiently connected. Anyone who has ever watched an infant get a shot at the doctor's office has probably noticed how long it takes for the baby to start crying afterward:

> The baby is happily smiling on the examining table when the doctor or nurse inserts the needle, depresses the plunger, and removes the needle. The baby is still smiling.
> Ten seconds pass, and the baby starts to look a bit perplexed.
> Another ten seconds pass, and the baby starts to look concerned.
> After another ten seconds, the baby begins to cry.

Nerve signals take a very long time to traverse a baby's tiny body. It takes quite a while for a baby to feel pain, and an even longer time to react to it.

Babies and young children also do not seem to feel physical pain as acutely as do older folks. For instance, infants are usually completely unfazed when they get bits of dirt, sawdust, fuzz, small insects, or eyelashes in their eyes. I have seen infants smiling and cooing and completely oblivious to foreign objects in their eyes, though those same foreign objects would induce excruciating agony in an adult eye.

When I was seven years old I injured my ankle in a jump-roping accident. My mother took me to the doctor, who refused to take an X-ray and sent us home. I ran around on that ankle for six months, until my mother noticed that I never put my right heel down on the ground when I walked. She took me to an orthopedist who took an X-ray and discovered that my ankle was broken. I was such an active child that I wore out two walking casts before I was healed.

I am pretty sure that no adult, including me, would be able to run around so blithely on a broken ankle for six months—the pain would be intolerable. When a child is sick or injured, it is important that the adults around her do not make assumptions about the amount of discomfort the child is feeling. It is quite likely that the child is not feeling as physically miserable as an adult would under the same circumstances.

Empathy is a very good thing, but in this instance it is probably misplaced and can induce adults to overmedicate children who are ill, or to unnecessarily upset children who are injured. If you have never witnessed this phenomenon, try spending some time at a playground and watch the way many children do not begin to cry immediately after they have hurt themselves; they often wait to begin wailing until they have reached a parent. (For information on solicitousness and pain in adults, see page 199.)

Though infants and children may not be very sensitive to physical pain and discomfort, they are exquisitely sensitive to emotional pain and suffering, both theirs and other people's. Thus it is much better for a child's physical and mental health if her parents are efficient and matter-of-fact when dealing with illnesses and injuries. If you pay more attention to children when they are injured or ill, you run a grave risk of turning them into hypochondriacs.

Little ones need enormous amounts of love; emotional pain hurts them far more than any physical injury ever could.

## NURSING INFANTS

A human infant acquires more than just nutrition when she nurses at her mother's breast. Many studies over the past two decades have shown that breast-feeding helps protect infants from respiratory infections, ear infections, diarrhea, gastrointestinal infections, bacterial meningitis, urinary tract infections, eczema, and asthma. Other studies have shown that children who were breast-fed as infants are less likely to be overweight or obese than are children who were fed formula.

## THE DESCENT OF HYPOCHONDRIA

Studies have shown that at least a quarter of all the patients sitting in doctors' offices report symptoms that seem to have no physical cause, and that one in ten patients who is tested for a terminal disease persists in believing he has a terminal disease even after the tests have proven him healthy. Though hypochondria may seem comical to those who are unaffected by the malady, in reality the disorder is disabling, expensive, and tends to run in families.

Charles Darwin, for example, was beset by heart pain and palpitations as he prepared to embark upon the *Beagle,* and wrote: "Like many an ignorant young man, especially one with a smattering of medical knowledge, I was convinced that I had heart disease. I did not consult any doctor, as I fully expected to hear the verdict that I was not fit for the voyage." Nevertheless, the *Beagle* set sail in December 1831 with Darwin on board.

In January 1839, Darwin married Emma Wedgwood. Their first son, William, was born eleven months later. Charles Darwin was almost constantly ill from the onset of his wife's first pregnancy until his death in 1882 at age seventy-three. The Darwins' union produced ten children, seven of whom lived to adulthood. Five of those survivors were described as hypochondriac, invalid, or depressed.

Charles Darwin's granddaughter, Gwen Raverat, in her memoir, *Period Piece*, wrote that her grandmother Emma "was a perfect nurse. She was like a rock to lean on, always devoted and unwearied in devising expedients to give relief, and neat handed and clever and carrying them out." But Raverat also wrote: "The trouble was that in my grandparents' house it was a distinction and a mournful pleasure to be ill. This was partly because my grandfather was always ill, and his children adored him and were inclined to imitate him; and partly because it was so delightful to be pitied and nursed by my grandmother. . . . I have sometimes thought that she must have been rather too sorry for her family when they were unwell. A little neglect . . . might have done them a world of good." Of her aunt Henrietta, Raverat wrote: "I have been told that when Aunt Etty was thirteen the doctor recommended, after she had a 'low fever,' that she should have breakfast in bed for a time. She never got up to breakfast again in all her life." Much later, when Henrietta was happily settled and married, "when there were colds about she often wore a kind of gas-mask of her own invention. It was an ordinary wire kitchen-strainer, stuffed with antiseptic cotton-wool, and tied on like a snout, with elastic over her ears. In this she would receive visitors and discuss politics in a hollow voice out of her eucalyptus-scented seclusion, oblivious of the fact that they might be struggling with fits of laughter."

A Finnish study that was published in the *American Journal of Clinical Nutrition* suggests that the types of bacteria living in a baby's gut may help determine whether that infant will become overweight or obese in later childhood. The researchers evaluated forty-nine children enrolled in a long-term study to evaluate the effects of probiotics on allergies. The children donated stool samples when they were six months old and then twelve months old. When the subjects reached the ripe old age of seven, the researchers selected twenty-five who were overweight or obese, and twenty-four who were of normal weight. The researchers then retrieved and analyzed the carefully stored baby poop samples. The slender children's samples contained twice as much probiotic bifidobacteria as the samples from the overweight children, while the heavy children's samples contained more *Staphylococcus aureus*. Researchers who analyzed samples of breast milk have found the following species of bifidobacteria in the samples: *Bifidobacterium longum*, *B. animalis*, *B. bifidum*, and *B. catenulatum*.

A 2003 study conducted by a team of social scientists from Purdue University and the University of Arizona showed that overweight children have an increased risk of becoming severely obese adults.

In the 1960s and 1970s, approximately 5 percent of American children were obese. The obesity index rose steadily after that, and finally reached a plateau: Between 1999 and 2006 a hefty 32 percent of our children were officially categorized as overweight or obese. Researchers are cautiously optimistic that the obesity index will not rise above its plateau.

## COUGH SYRUP

Some members of the American College of Chest Physicians reviewed decades' worth of studies and concluded that there is no scientific evidence whatsoever that the active ingredients in most over-the-counter cough medicines—dextromethorphan, a cough suppressant, and guaifenesin, an expectorant—have any effect at all on coughs. The doctors did find, however, that over-the-counter cough medicines have a very strong placebo effect.

In 2007, the Centers for Disease Control and Prevention (CDC) announced that over a two-year period, fifteen hundred toddlers and babies were treated in emergency rooms because of bad reactions to cold or cough medicine; three of these infants died. After the CDC's announcement, the pharmaceutical industry voluntarily withdrew all "infant" cough medications from the market. Also in 2007, the Food and Drug Administration warned parents that cough and cold medicines should never be given to children under the age of two, and advised against giving them to children under the age of six.

According to a spokesman for the maker of Robitussin products, quoted in USA Today: "Our stance is that the FDA has reviewed dextromethorphan and guaifenesin and found the two ingredients to be both safe and effective. We don't believe that consumers would . . . re-purchase these products if they weren't efficacious."

## A SPOONFUL OF HONEY

Ian M. Paul, M.D., led a study on 105 children between the ages of two and eighteen who had upper respiratory tract infections. One group of children was dosed with honey, another group was given dextromethorphan, and the last group was not given anything for their coughs. The researchers found that honey helped reduce the cough frequency and severity, and improved both the children's and the parents' sleep; dextromethorphan did not.

Note: *Never, never, never* give honey to infants who are less than a year old! Infants' tiny, immature digestive systems lack the enzymes that break down the botulism spores commonly found in honey. When swallowed by an infant, the spores activate and start producing toxins. The resulting botulism is frequently fatal. (Hummingbirds are also susceptible to honey-induced botulism. Never use honey to make nectar for your hummingbird feeder.)

## BACTERIAL INFECTIONS, BACTERIAL INJECTIONS

In the 1890s, a New York surgeon named William Coley began testing a new treatment: He would treat his terminally ill bone cancer patients by injecting them with pathogenic bacteria. Unfortunately, the injections killed a couple of his first patients. Coley then changed his tactics and began inject-ing his patients either with large numbers of heat-killed bacteria or with the toxins produced by bacteria, neither of which can cause infection, in order to avoid actually infecting his patients. After suffering through weeks of fever and chills, his patients recovered from the bacterial injections, and many of their tumors shrank.

Dr. Coley had been inspired to try this drastic treatment after one of his first patients, a seventeen-year-old girl, rapidly died of bone cancer. In despair, Coley combed through the literature and found many reports of severe infections that had caused malignant tumors to regress or disappear. Coley's work was not universally applauded in his day.

In the 1980s, dermatologists began noticing that patients who had severe acne, which is caused by bacteria, had lower than average rates of skin cancer, lymphoma, and leukemia. And studies show that cotton and livestock workers, who are constantly breathing large amounts of bacteria-laden dust, have a reduced risk of lung cancer.

Harvey Checkoway, an epidemiologist at the University of Washing-ton, Seattle, has found that female cotton workers in Shanghai are 40 to 60 percent less likely to develop cancer of the lung, breast, or pancreas than are their less dusty counterparts, and Giuseppe Mastrangelo of the University of Padua in Italy found that Italian dairy farmers who are exposed to high levels of manure dust have only one-fifth the risk of developing lung cancer as do their peers who work in less dusty open fields.

These researchers believe that the protective effect of dust is due to the body's reaction to the endotoxins produced by bacteria that live in the dust. But Checkoway does not recommend dust-sniffing as a panacea, because though the dairy farmers and cotton workers have a reduced risk of cancer, they tend to have high rates of other respiratory problems.

Researchers are studying the effectiveness of injecting cancerous tumors with bacteria that have been heat-killed or that have been rendered harmless through genetic manipulation. Dr. John Stanford, a researcher at Univer-sity College, London, believes that exposure to endotoxins encourages the immune system to switch its tactics, so that rather than sending out antibod-ies, which are ineffectual at killing cancer, it begins sending out white blood cells, which are actually capable of engulfing and killing cancer cells.

## SNOT FOR TOTS

Studies conducted in the 1970s showed that patients who had Hodgkin's disease (a cancer of the lymphatic system) tended to come from high-income, well-educated families who lived in the suburbs, and that people who had fewer siblings had a higher risk of developing Hodgkin's. In 2004, Ellen Chang, a researcher at the Harvard School of Public Health, analyzed the case histories of 565 people with Hodgkin's disease and 679 control subjects. She was expecting similar findings from her study, but she found no correlation between socioeconomic status and Hodgkin's. There was, however, an association with day care attendance: People who had attended day care for a year or more were 36 percent less likely to develop Hodgkin's disease than were those who had never been in day care. That study led to another study of the impact of growing up with multiple siblings, which showed that people who grew up in a family with several older siblings were less likely to develop Hodgkin's disease than were those who grew up with fewer siblings.

Chang believes that early infections can "prime" the immature immune system, and this more experienced, robust immune system provides greater protection against bacterial and viral infection in later life.

One of the more common viruses that children tend to swap around is the Epstein-Barr virus, which causes either a mild illness or no symptoms at all in young children, but often causes mononucleosis in adolescents and young adults. Because this disease is transmitted by exposure to saliva, mono is somewhat jokingly referred to as "the kissing disease" when it strikes adolescents. Unfortunately, epidemiological studies have shown that people who have had mononucleosis are three times more likely to get Hodgkin's disease than are those who have never had mononucleosis. What does this mean? Should we all refuse to kiss each other? Not at all, keep kissing: 95 percent of all adults between the ages of thirty-five and forty already have antibodies against the Epstein-Barr virus, though most people catch the virus while still young enough to avoid serious illness. We lucky ones don't remember having "mono" because we caught the Epstein-Barr virus when we were three and then had a runny nose for a couple of days. Mononucleosis is much more memorable because it causes, among other things: sore throat, fever, headaches, muscle aches, abdominal pain, and swollen glands.

Mono's acute phase can last up to a month, and it may take three months for the patient to get fully back to normal.

Once caught, the Epstein-Barr virus becomes a permanent resident of the body, remaining mostly dormant, but with occasional flare-ups. There are usually no symptoms and no feeling of malaise during these flare-ups, but the active virus can be spread to others. In other words, you can catch the Epstein-Barr virus from almost anyone, even from someone who has no symptoms at all, and you are much better off if you catch the virus early in life! So let those toddlers slobber on each other, share each other's ice cream cones and lollipops, and make mud pies with dirt and spit. Everyone will end up much healthier.


## RISK

For several decades, our society has been trying to keep our children as safe as possible, removing playground equipment that is considered too dangerous, such as teeter-totters; tall swings, slides, and monkey bars; and just about everything else that used to make playgrounds fun. We are terrified of what the FBI terms "stereotypical kidnappings," which it defines as "abductions perpetrated by a stranger or slight acquaintance and involving a child who was transported 50 or more miles, detained overnight, held for ransom or with the intent to keep the child permanently, or killed." We try to protect our children by keeping them indoors. We prevent them from being independent by building neighborhoods and shopping areas without sidewalks. The result has been an unprecedented epidemic of childhood obesity and asthma.

FBI statistics show that there were 115 "stereotypical child kidnappings" in 2002. But nearly 5 million American children suffer from asthma, and they suffer every year, all year long. American Lung Association statistics show that in 2002, asthma killed 170 children younger than 15 years of age; sent approximately 640,000 children to the emergency room; and caused American youngsters to miss a combined total of 12.8 million days of school.

In 2006, nearly a third of American children were either overweight or obese. Overweight children are likely to remain overweight for the rest of their lives, and because of this excess weight, their lives may be plagued with chronic diseases that are associated with excess weight.

Coddling is a great way to prepare eggs but a terrible way to prepare children.

## BRAVE GREEN CHILDREN

How brave should we be on behalf of our children? Do parents have the right, or the obligation, to make their children suffer in the here and now in the hope that they may reap the benefits in the future? As they say, "no pain, no gain," but it can be difficult to watch one's precious little one screaming in pain or fear at the doctor's office before, during, or after vaccination.

The spectacular success of childhood vaccinations in preventing once ubiquitous and terrifying childhood diseases such as polio, measles, mumps, whooping cough, chicken pox, and diphtheria has made many parents fear the possible side effects of vaccines more than they fear the diseases themselves. If you have never experienced any of these childhood diseases yourself, and you have never encountered anyone else who has, the slight risk of complications due to the vaccine may seem intolerable. Luckily for most of the parents who decide not to vaccinate their own precious offspring, there is such a thing as "herd immunity," a phenomenon that helps protect even uninoculated children from contracting diseases as long as they are surrounded by large numbers of children who have been inoculated. In communities with large numbers of children who have gotten all their "baby shots," there is indeed a relatively low risk that uninoculated children will contract these diseases. But if a large percentage of a community's precious children have not been inoculated, the herd immunity breaks down. Uninoculated children can spread diseases to children who have been inoculated but whose immune systems did not react strongly enough to afford them complete protection, as well as to children who are too young to have gotten their full complement of shots.

From the beginning, the idea of inoculation has frequently met with great resistance, sometimes with violent resistance. Colonial America was ravaged approximately once every ten years by a smallpox epidemic that decimated the population and terrified the populace. But when a smallpox epidemic broke out in Boston in 1721, Cotton Mather, a prominent Puritan minister, was informed by his African-born slave, Onesimus, about an inoculation procedure that had been practiced in Africa for centuries. The procedure utilized fresh, infective material that had been extracted from the smallpox pustule of an infected person; a thorn was then used to scratch the pus into the skin of an uninfected person. Cotton Mather convinced a doctor named Zabdiel Boylston to attempt the procedure. Boylston vaccinated his own son, Tommy, and then two of his slaves, a father and son named Jack and Jackey. The three subjects developed mild symptoms, then recovered. Many people, both in the colonies and in the Old World, had violently objected to vaccination, saying it was unnatural and subverted God's will, and Mather's and Boylston's lives were threatened. Despite the threat of violence, Boylston managed to inoculate a total of 244 people against smallpox. Six (nearly 2.5 percent) of these volunteers died. A total of 5,980 uninoculated people came down with smallpox during the epidemic, and 844 (more than 14 percent) of them died.

In 1980, as a result of a massive, relentless, worldwide program of smallpox vaccination, the World Health Organization was able to declare that the scourge of smallpox had been completely eradicated from the face of the earth.

## CHILDHOOD DISEASES

Before the advent of the measles vaccine, there were approximately 400,000 cases of the measles each year in the United States. There are still many parts of the world in which children are not routinely vaccinated against measles. But worldwide, measles fatalities fell by 60 percent between 1999, when there were an estimated 873,000 deaths, and 2005, when there were 345,000. This improvement was largely due to enormous progress in vaccinating children in Africa.

Even if measles does not kill a child, it can still maim her. Complications of measles include ear infections, diarrhea, secondary bronchitis or pneumonia, and encephalitis, which can cause brain damage or death. Undernourished children in developing countries are particularly suscep- tible to measles-induced blindness, and between 15,000 and 60,000 of these innocents lose their sight each year.

Many parents who opt out of getting their children vaccinated are afraid that vaccines, or thimerosal (a mercury-based preservative that was commonly added to vaccines), cause autism. Thimerosal was banned from vaccines in Denmark in 1992. A study of the relationship between thimerosal and autism was led by Kreesten M. Madsen, M.D., of the Department of Epidemiology and Social Medicine at the University of Aarhus. Her team analyzed the records of all psychiatric admissions in Denmark between 1971 and 2000, as well as all outpatient contacts in psychiatric departments in Denmark between 1995 and 2000. They saw no increase in the incidence of autism from 1971 through 1990, but "From 1991 until 2000 the incidence increased and continued to rise after the removal of thimerosal from vaccines, including increases among children born after the discontinuation of thimerosal. . . . The discontinuation of thimerosal-containing vaccines in Denmark in 1992 was followed by an increase in the incidence of autism. Our ecological data do not support a correlation between thimerosal-containing vaccines and the incidence of autism."

If we want to jump to a hasty conclusion about the relationship between vaccinations and autism, perhaps we should opine that a lack of exposure to thimerosal causes autism!

In Philadelphia in 1991, a religious group that did not believe in vac- cinations was the epicenter of a measles outbreak that killed 8 and sickened more than 700 people. Most of the victims were children.

In 1999–2000, a measles epidemic in the Netherlands sickened 3,292 people, only 1 of whom had been fully vaccinated. Three children, ages two, three, and seventeen, died, 72 others were hospitalized, and 16 percent of all the measles patients had complications. Unvaccinated individuals were up to 460 times more likely to contract measles than were those who had been vaccinated.

According to the World Health Organization, if measles vaccinations were stopped entirely, they would expect 2.7 million measles fatalities each year.

Pertussis (whooping cough) is another disease that most people have not experienced, but according to the CDC, before the first pertussis vaccine became widely available in the 1940s, there were between 150,000 and 260,000 cases of whooping cough in the United States every year. Up to 9,000 of these cases were fatal. In the early 1980s, many parents began refusing to have their children vaccinated, and the annual number of pertussis cases has been increasing ever since. From 1990 to 1996, 57 people died in the United States from pertussis, and 49 of those victims were less than six months old.

I have had direct experience with pertussis: Over a decade ago, I developed (and practiced, and perfected) prolonged bouts of coughing that gave me two black eyes and left me gasping for breath. I went to the doctor, who informed me that he thought I had whooping cough. This was years before the experts had figured out that the pertussis vaccine eventually wears off. My exhausting, weeks-long experience with whooping cough made me understand why so many babies and small children succumb to the disease. I was lucky that I had a mild case—some whooping cough sufferers cough until they vomit (dozens of times a day), while others cough so hard they break ribs. Now there is a pertussis booster shot for adults. According to Dr. Mark Dworkin, of the Division of Epidemiology and Biostatistics at the University of Illinois at the Chicago School of Public Health, "we need to use the newly available booster vaccines against pertussis for adults and adolescents widely because this may get pertussis back under control. Adults and adolescents can get coughing illness that may last for weeks or even months and they represent a large reservoir of infection, putting others, such as vulnerable infants, at increased risk of infection."

Diphtheria is a bacterial disease that used to strike terror into the hearts of parents. In 1921, there were 205,000 cases of diphtheria in the United States, and 15,520 of the patients died. The first diphtheria vaccine was developed in 1923, and cases in the United States dropped off sharply after that, though the disease is still common in other parts of the world. For instance, after the breakup of the Soviet Union, the public health system broke down, vaccination levels dropped, and between 1990 and 1999, there were more than 150,000 reported cases of diphtheria and 5,000 deaths reported in the former Soviet Union.

Mark Twain wrote a short story called "Experience of the McWilliamses with Membranous Croup" in 1875. (In Twain's day, diphtheria was known as membranous croup.) The account is simultaneously funny, loving, and touching. If you would like to gain an inkling of what it was like for devoted parents when an epidemic struck their town, I strongly suggest that you hunt this story down and devour it.

Rubella (German measles) is a disease that is usually quite mild and almost innocuous to those who have already been born, but causes terrible birth defects in children whose mothers contract the disease while pregnant. Up to 90 percent of children whose mothers contracted rubella during the first trimester of pregnancy develop problems such as heart defects, cataracts, mental retardation, deafness, or cerebral palsy. (One of my childhood friends had birth defects because her mother had caught German measles while pregnant. She was born with hydrocephaly, a pair of knees that barely bent, a nonopposable thumb on her right hand, and cerebral palsy. She used crutches and considered herself very lucky because she was not wheelchair-bound.)

The rubella vaccine is one of the few vaccines that is intended to protect someone other than the person who is being stuck with the needle. We are all in this together, folks!

## THE KINDEST CUT?

There is another minor medical intervention that protects more than just the person undergoing the procedure: neonatal circumcision. I have been watching the research on this topic for several years now, and it has been illuminating.

## EGYPTIAN SURGERY

The Edwin Smith Surgical Papyrus, which dates from the seventeenth century B.C., contains forty-eight systematically organized case studies. Egyptian medicine was quite sophisticated, and the Surgical Papyrus describes treating crushing head injuries, stitching up wounds, setting broken bones, and poulticing infected wounds; it also noted which types of wounds could not be treated. The Edwin Smith Surgical Papyrus documents Egyptian doctors' observation that a certain percentage of baby boys were born with foreskins so tight that they prevented urination (the modern term for this condition is phimosis). The treatment for this condition was circumcision.

There is no way of knowing what percentage of baby boys born in ancient Egypt had phimosis, but in 1953, Colonel T. E. Osmond, M.B., a doctor with the Royal Army Medical Corps in Great Britain, found that 35 percent of uncircumcised soldiers would have "benefitted from circumcision" due to hygiene problems, and 14 percent of uncircumcised soldiers "needed circumcision" because they were in pain or suffering from sexual dysfunction and/or urination problems that were caused by deformities of the foreskin.

Colonel Osmond did not elaborate upon exactly what these soldiers were suffering from, but the foreskin is, and apparently always has been, prone to a host of ailments that include: phimosis, balanitis (chronic dermatitis and inflammation), and paraphimosis, which occurs when the foreskin is left in a retracted position, cutting off circulation and causing swelling and fluid retention. Paraphimosis is considered a urological emergency; if it is not treated, gangrene or autoamputation of the penis may ensue.

The ancient Egyptians practiced circumcision in order to improve health and hygiene, and the procedure was adopted as a religious practice by the ancient Jews and then by Muslims. Circumcision was fairly uncommon among non-Jews and non-Muslims in the United States until the beginning of the twentieth century, when it became much more common. In the last couple of decades, however, there has been a swing in the other direction, as more parents decided to leave their boys intact. The arguments against circumcision revolve around the psychological trauma involved, the right of the individual to determine what happens to his own body, the desire to avoid inflicting pain on infants, and wanting to avoid having babies associate pain with their parents.

Many anticircumcision websites feature testimonials from circumcised men who apparently felt deep rage, sadness, and hate because they were circumcised against their will when they were infants. Here are a few quotes from one such website:

"Circumcision has given my life a much diminished and shameful flavor."

"The single most traumatic event of my life with the greatest psychological damage was my circumcision as an infant."

"Circumcision, it's taught me how to hate."

"Being circumcised has ruined my sex life." (One may well ask about someone who was circumcised as an infant: "How does he know?")

"I feel violated and abused."

"I have felt unhappy about it all my life."

"I am very angry and resentful about this. I've had many physical, psychological, and emotional problems all my life."

"I feel cheated at having been robbed of what is my natural birthright."

And last, but not least: "I feel like the best part of me was severed from my body, and I have ugly scars to remind me. I am so ANGRY!"

Many of these anticircumcisionists have the audacity to compare male circumcision with female circumcision. Anyone who could seriously compare the two practices is definitely not paying attention. Male circumcision is like removing the wart from the tip of someone's nose. Female circumcision is like removing the entire nose along with the wart, and then sewing the open sinuses shut with fresh, unsterilized catgut.

Female "circumcision" is actually complete amputation and mutilation done with very crude instruments under dangerously unsanitary conditions. The procedure confers no benefits whatsoever, but rather causes pain and endangers the victim's life and health during the operation as well as ever afterward. On the other hand, there is quite a lot of evidence that routine, neonatal male circumcision does confer substantial health benefits.

In contrast, there are quite a few websites where men who were circumcised as adults write about their experiences, and all the contributors seem quite pleased with the results and pleased with themselves. In fact, they are so graphically pleased that their comments are completely unsuitable for inclusion in a book that will not be shipped in a plain brown wrapper.

Male circumcision confers health benefits not only upon the recipient, but also on his sex partners. It has been known for many years that the wives and/or sexual partners of circumcised men are far less likely to get cervical cancer than are the wives of uncircumcised men, and recent studies have revealed many more health benefits.

## PROTECTING WOMEN

Studies conducted by Johns Hopkins researchers in Uganda, and published in 2006, showed that male circumcision reduced the AIDS transmission rate between HIV-positive men and their uninfected female partners by 30 percent. During the study, 299 women contracted HIV from uncircumcised partners, while only 44 women were infected by circumcised men.

The study confirmed anecdotal evidence from Africa that had shown that regions in which circumcision is common had lower rates of HIV infection than did areas in which circumcision was uncommon.

A clinical trial in South Africa also showed that circumcised men are less likely to contract AIDS from HIV-positive women.

According to the researchers, the inner lining of the foreskin is made up of cells that bind to the AIDS virus much more easily than do the cells that comprise the other parts of the penis. Removal of the foreskin may simply reduce the amount of exposure to the HIV virus.

## AFRICAN TRUCKERS, A VIRUS'S BEST FRIENDS

A study conducted by researchers from the United States and Kenya, and published in the February 15, 2005, issue of the *Journal of Infectious Diseases*, calculated the probability of HIV infection for men who have multiple, concurrent heterosexual partners. The research subjects were male Kenyan truckers, who are apparently so extraordinarily promiscuous that their travels were largely responsible for the rapid spread of the HIV virus across the African continent.

Between 1993 and 1997, a total of 745 HIV-negative male truckers based in Mombasa, Kenya, participated in a study. These volunteers were asked to give information about the number of sexual encounters they had and with whom: wives, casual partners, or prostitutes. During the course of the study, the participants were screened for HIV and other sexually transmitted diseases.

The researchers excluded men whose ethnic or cultural differences made their sexual habits different from the Kenyan truckers' norm. Uncircumcised men in this study had a one in eighty chance of becoming infected with the HIV virus each time they had sex, while the circumcised men had a one in two hundred chance of becoming infected with HIV each time they had sex.

## PROTECTING MEN

Another clinical trial conducted in Africa, this one by scientists from the University of Illinois at Chicago, was halted prematurely by the National Institutes of Health (NIH) in December 2006 because preliminary results showed that circumcision reduces heterosexual men's risk of contracting the HIV virus by 53 percent. The NIH recommended that all men in the study who remained uncircumcised be offered circumcision. "Circumcision is now a proven, effective prevention strategy to reduce HIV infections in men," said the principal investigator of the study, Robert Bailey, professor of epidemiology at the University of Illinois at Chicago School of Public Health.

Researchers had enrolled 2,784 uncircumcised volunteers, all of whom were HIV-negative, between the ages of eighteen and twenty-four, and lived in Kisumu, Kenya. (The researchers chose to work in Kisumu because an estimated 26 percent of the uncircumcised men in the region are HIV-positive by the age of twenty-five.) Half the volunteers were randomly assigned to be circumcised. All the participants received free HIV testing and counseling, condoms, behavioral risk counseling, medical care, and tests and treatments for sexually transmitted diseases, for twenty-four months.

During the study, 22 of the 1,393 circumcised men contracted HIV, compared to 47 of the 1,391 uncircumcised men.

Kevin De Cock, M.D., the director of the World Health Organization's HIV/AIDS program, was quoted as saying that male circumcision could avert as many as two million new HIV infections over the course of a decade in sub-Saharan Africa alone. Ethics boards later halted two more studies, when similar research in Uganda and Kenya showed AIDS reduction rates of more than 50 percent for circumcised males.

Testing of an HIV vaccine being developed by Merck was halted in September 2007 after a safety monitoring committee determined that the vaccine had failed in both of its main objectives. The vaccine had failed to prevent new HIV infections, and had also failed to lower the blood levels of HIV virus among participants who became infected. The results from three thousand participants in nine countries also suggested that the vaccine might have increased the risk of HIV infection. Scientific analysis found that the highest risk of HIV infection among recipients of the Merck vaccine was in uncircumcised males who had preexisting antibodies to the adenovirus type-5 that was used to produce the vaccine. (Adenoviruses are a group of viruses that commonly cause upper respiratory infections such as the common cold, croup, pneumonia, and bronchitis.)

A study headed by Aaron A. R. Tobian, M.D., Ph.D., in Uganda, followed nearly 3,400 men who were negative for HSV-2, the virus that causes genital herpes. After two years, the researchers concluded that circumcised men have a 25 percent lower risk of contracting genital herpes.

## WHAT ABOUT YOUR BABY? WHAT'S IN IT FOR HIM?

Even males who do not live in sub-Saharan Africa benefit from circumcision:

1. Studies have shown that uncircumcised infants have ten to twelve times more urinary tract infections than do their circumcised peers.
2. Cervical cancer is the second most common cancer in women worldwide, and almost all cases may be caused by the human papillomavirus (HPV). It has been known for many years that the female partners of men who are circumcised are less likely to get cervical cancer than are women whose partners are uncircumcised. (I would like to think that men benefit from not giving their partners cancer!)
3. A study conducted in Spain, Colombia, Brazil, Thailand, and the Philippines between 1985 and 1993 showed that the circumcised men in the study were 60 percent less likely to be harboring the HPV virus than were uncircumcised men. Perhaps not coincidentally, the study also found that the odds of cervical cancer were reduced by about 60 percent in women whose partners were circumcised.

4. Infection with the human papillomavirus increases the risk of invasive penile cancer, a potentially lethal disease with a five-year
survival rate of 65 percent in the United States. A 1991 review
of 592 invasive penile cancer cases from five major cancer centers
in the United States included no men who had been circumcised
in infancy, despite the fact that more than half the baby boys
born in the United States by the mid-1930s were circumcised,
and by the 1960s, more than 80 percent of American baby boys
were circumcised. Over a fifty-five-year period, more than 50,000
American men were diagnosed with invasive penile cancer, and
only 10 of those men had been circumcised as infants.

The authors of a study of invasive penile cancer conducted at the
Research Division of the Kaiser Permanente Medical Care Program in Oakland, California, estimated the lifetime risk of invasive penile cancer for an
uncircumcised American male at one in six hundred. Men who were circumcised after the neonatal period still have an elevated risk compared to
those who were circumcised as newborns. The cure for the most severe cases
of invasive penile cancer is penectomy, or total amputation.

## TOUGH GUYS

Neonatal circumcision may lower a male's sensitivity to pain in later life.

Wendy Sternberg, Ph.D., of Haverford College in Pennsylvania, has
been conducting research on mice that suggests that an adult's pain tolerance may be directly linked to the animal's prior exposure to pain and stress.

According to Sternberg: "Recent medical advances allow potentially
painful procedures such as surgery to be performed on infants just hours old,
or in some cases, even in the womb." In order to learn about the effects of
such early exposure to pain, Sternberg and her colleagues performed abdominal surgery on forty newborn mice. The researchers anesthetized the skin,
cut an incision, probed inside, then closed the wound back up. Twenty of
these mice were given morphine for postoperative pain relief, and the other
twenty were given a saltwater solution (which gives no pain relief). A group

of mice that had not been operated on were given either morphine or salt solution, and served as a control group.

When the tiny participants matured, they were given a series of tests that measured their pain response. The mice that had been operated on but had not been given any postoperative pain treatment were less sensitive to pain than were all the other mice in the study. The researchers concluded that the effects were due to the experience of pain associated with the surgery, rather than to the surgery itself or the anesthesia.

It is possible that infants who are circumcised may grow into men who are better able to tolerate pain. High tolerance to pain can be a very good thing! No one likes to see a baby crying, but sometimes a little pain in the here and now can yield large benefits in the future. Lest anyone mistake my intentions, I am not advocating for compulsory circumcision, I just want parents of newborn boys to be able to make truly informed decisions.

I recently read a blog written by the mother of a baby boy. In it she noted that her son had had to be circumcised when he was three months old: "my baby got Phimosis because the foreskin fully unable to retract and he unable to urinate. So the last option was circumcision."

This information set off a wave of outrage. Among the comments: "What!?!? There is no such thing as phimosis in a 3 month old baby. Most boy's foreskins don't retract till they are 5–10 years old. Even in cases of genuine phimosis (which is rare), circumcision should be an absolute last resort. It can almost always be treated without surgery."

And another: "After reading the excuses/reasons for circumcising a newborn male infant the only conclusion that I can come to is that it's a slap in the face for Nature/God. Your action says to 'Nature/God' that your design of the male genitalia is flawed and I have corrected it. All males including animals were given a foreskin for a reason. Recent research in Michigan has shown that naturally intact men have much more feeling and sensitivity in their penis than altered (Circumcised) men. It would of been nice if had given your son a chance to find out what nature had intended for him."

Note: These are exact quotes. The grammatical errors are exactly as they appeared in the original postings.

I can't help wondering what about "he unable to urinate" these outraged people didn't get? I would like to believe that Nature/God never makes mistakes, but I have experienced and witnessed enough of them myself to know otherwise. There are indeed such things as birth defects that affect the male reproductive system, and many of these birth defects are caused by man-made chemicals. What "Nature/God" intended for the baby in question was probably an early death caused by an inability to urinate.

And a final note for the insatiably curious: What happens to the foreskin after it is removed from the baby?

If the parents give their consent, some foreskins are sold to laboratories, where they are used in AIDS research, because those tiny bits of unwanted tissue are the most effective known culture medium for the HIV virus. Foreskins that are not sold to laboratories are discarded at the hospital.

## LITTLE GREEN BARBARIANS

When your child sees that you are afraid to touch anything, anywhere, and anytime, you are teaching him that the world is a dangerous place, that seemingly harmless, inanimate objects may kill or harm him at any time, and that he is too delicate to survive in our world. If you do this very earnestly, you may well make it come true. Fear is a powerful emotion, and it changes the way our bodies work.

Our son was an extremely oral child who was frequently discovered sucking his dirty socks (while they were on his feet), sucking seat backs in train or bus stations, and licking windows in public places. We certainly did not encourage these behaviors, but these things happen. Perhaps as a direct consequence of his unsanitary early behavior, our son was, and is, almost never sick, is allergic to nothing, and is afraid of almost nothing. Maybe we should all suck more socks.

# In Conclusion

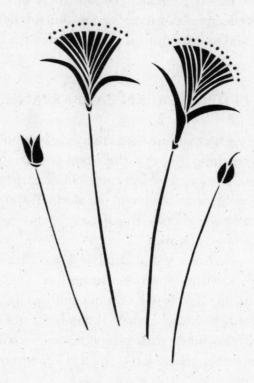

## TAKE A RISK

The maggot therapy website contains the following exchange: "I think I ate a maggot. Will I die?" A very wise maggot expert replied: "Yes, eventually; but probably not as a result of the maggot."

Newton's Third Law of Motion states that for every action there is an equal and opposite reaction. Life is like that, too. If you try to tightly control your life in order to reduce a specific risk, the risk of something else is almost sure to increase. We take risks all the time, whether we are aware of them or not. Some risks are just more fun than others. We might as well choose risks that are fun, creative, productive, profitable, or life-enhancing. There is no way to learn from your mistakes until you make a few. Playing it safe isn't really playing, is it?

My previous book, *Organic Housekeeping*, was meant to function as an encyclopedic resource for householders. Much to my astonishment, several people have asked whether I actually do all these chores on a regular basis. The answer is a resounding and somewhat hysterical *no!* Though I tested as many of the techniques as I could, given the limitations of my decidedly unpalatial house, which suffers from an appalling lack of marble floors, silver tea services, gold tableware, diamond jewelry, crystal chandeliers, real linen bedsheets, silken draperies, and Louis XIV furniture. I do not, cannot, and will not perform the vast majority of these tasks on an ongoing basis, because I simply do not give a damn about "gracious living." I care deeply about the health and happiness of my family and friends. I care deeply about the environment. And as far as my housekeeping goes (which generally isn't far): The people who matter to me don't mind, and the people who mind don't matter.

Long, long ago, when I was an art student in college, my watercolor professor told us that we were each to produce an icon for that week's assignment. He talked about icons, showed some slides of icons, and talked about their meaning. We were to think about the assignment and do a watercolor of what we considered sacred.

I thought hard, and came to the conclusion that the most iconic, most sacred object in America was the dollar bill. I sketched out my ideas, and then went to the art store to buy some imitation gold leaf and some compatible glue.

I chose a nice, clean, crisp one-dollar bill, carefully cut it up, then rearranged it so that it formed a Madonna and Child. The eye in the pyramid formed the Child's head. Like a buffalo hunter, I wasted nothing—every single piece of that dollar bill was used as a design element. I carefully marked where all the components went, then moved the pieces out of the way so I could paint the background in glowing, iconic colors. I allowed the paper to dry, then glued on the Madonna and Child; when they stabilized, I added the "gold leaf" halos and stars. When the thing was done, it was rather pretty.

I brought my icon to class the next week, and pinned it up on the wall with the other icons to be critiqued.

My icon nearly caused a riot. All the other students were furious with me. Most of their comments ran along these lines: "Here I am struggling to get by and she's cutting up dollar bills!" But the materials for that tiny icon, including the dollar bill, cost far less than the materials for the large watercolors most of us usually brought to the class. Apparently, I had desecrated an icon in order to make an icon.

Just as you have to break some eggs in order to make an omelette, you have to use some materials to make an art piece. There is no such thing as a zero-impact life. No matter what we do or don't do, we affect the planet. But if we are mindful of what we are doing, our overall impact can be positive rather than negative.

The idea of a pristine wilderness that is completely free of human impact is romantic, but it exists nowhere on earth. The seemingly untrammeled American landscape that European explorers first encountered was actually the product of sophisticated land management practiced by the indigenous people. These original inhabitants used fire to manage and maintain ecosystems that could produce healthy populations of elk, deer, bison, and bear. The open prairies in the center of the continent and the parklike forests of the east were created by these first people. When the gardeners disappeared, their garden deteriorated.

Even the wild, exotic Amazon jungle is largely the product of human intervention; that is why it more closely resembles an orchard than it does an untrammeled wilderness. In some areas, nearly half of the environmentally important plant species are species that are used by humans. Many researchers believe that this incredibly diverse ecosystem is a work of human artifice right down through the topsoil, and has been managed by human beings for millennia.

At the end of the nineteenth century, explorers in the Amazon noticed deposits of dark, extremely fertile soil that were as much as two meters deep, which the locals referred to as *terra preta do Indio* (Indian black earth).

When twentieth-century researchers finally began studying the phenomenon, they realized that patches of terra preta were surrounded by the extremely poor, and sometimes even toxic, soils that are the norm in the Amazonian rain forest. Terra preta is riddled with charcoal and contains shards of millennia-old ceramics; the researchers realized that both these materials had been purposefully incorporated into the soil. Apparently the original inhabitants believed that when life hands you impoverished, unproductive soils, you should make terra preta!

Tests that compared terra preta to the surrounding soils showed that terra preta is richer in plant-available phosphorus, calcium, sulfur, and nitrogen. It also contains much more organic matter, retains moisture and nutrients more readily, and has much higher populations of soil microbes than the surrounding soil. Terra preta's carbon levels also proved to be at least five times higher than the levels found in the surrounding soils. Many researchers now believe that carbon-rich soils are sequestering huge amounts of carbon that might otherwise be circulating in the atmosphere and contributing to global warming.

Étienne Dambrine, of the National Institute for Agronomic Research in Champenoux, France, studied the environmental effects of 108 Roman settlements that were excavated in the Tronçais forest. Before the discovery of these Roman settlements, people had assumed that the forest, which is famous for its magnificent oak trees and plentiful wildlife, was pristine and relatively untouched by human beings. Dambrine and his colleagues discovered that the plant and animal life was much more diverse and abundant in areas where the ancient Romans farmed. The researchers attributed this richness to ancient Roman fertilization practices. Dambrine and his colleagues wrote: "Latin authors repeatedly mention the need for regular fertilization after plowing, using ashes or animal manure. Domestic garbage, including some broken ceramics, was redistributed with manure and ashes." The researchers believed that the chemical changes caused by such activity might be "irreversible."

This is the Garden of Eden, and we are still the gardeners. It's time to roll up our sleeves and get back to work.

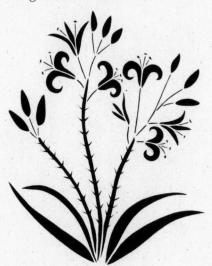

# Acknowledgments

This book would not have been possible without support, assistance, input, advice, and help from the following people:

Dmitri Sandbeck, Nick Tramdack, and Glenn Gordon—patient and wise readers, editors, and researchers

Anne Berne, Suzanne Seeley, and Constance Dretske—patient and helpful readers

Tisse Takagi—Jane Austen research

Ariadne Sandbeck—French translation

Tim Kaiser and Carolyn Olson—technology assistance

Jean Sramek and Susie Newman—food consultants

Ann Klefstad—grammatical consultant

Al and Lynda Parella and Charlie Nichol—chemical consultants

Janis Donnaud—world's best literary agent

Whitney Frick—editor

Walt Sandbeck—light and love of my life

Thank you!

# Bibliography

### Books

Ashenburg, Katherine. *The Dirt on Clean: An Unsanitized History*. New York: North Point Press, a division of Farrar, Straus & Giroux, 2007.

Balsdon, J. P. V. D. *Life and Leisure in Ancient Rome*. New York: McGraw-Hill Book Company, 1969.

Bayard, Tania, translator and editor. *A Medieval Home Companion: Housekeeping in the Fourteenth Century*. New York: HarperPerennial, a division of HarperCollins Publishers, 1991.

Beecher, Catherine. *A Treatise on Domestic Economy*. Boston: Thomas Webb & Co., 1843.

Belote, Julianne. *The Compleat American Housewife 1776*. Concord, Calif.: Nitty Gritty Productions, 1974.

Budge, E. A. Wallis. *Literature of the Ancient Egyptians*. London: J. M. Dent & Sons Ltd., 1914.

Callahan, Gerald N. *Infection: The Uninvited Universe*. New York: St. Martin's Press, 2006.

Castiglione, Baldassare. *The Courtyer; Very necessary and profitable for yonge Gentilmen and Gentilwomen abiding in Court, Palace, or Place. Done into Englyshe by Thomas Hoby*. London: Essex House Press, 1900.

Cowell, F. R. *Everyday Life in Ancient Rome*. London: B. T. Batsford Ltd.; New York: G. P. Putnam's Sons, 1961.

Deming, W. Edwards. *Out of the Crisis*. Cambridge, Mass.: MIT Press, 1982.

Duncan, David Douglas. *The Private World of Pablo Picasso*. New York: Ridge Press, 1958.

Durant, Will. *The Story of Civilization*, Part 1: *Our Oriental Heritage*. New York: Simon & Schuster, 1954.

Dyer, Betsey Dexter. *A Field Guide to Bacteria*. Ithaca, N.Y.: Cornell University Press, 2003.

Eighner, Lars. *Travels with Lizbeth: Three Years on the Road and on the Streets*. New York: St. Martin's Press, 1993.

Erickson, Laura. *101 Ways to Help Birds*. Mechanicsburg, Pa.: Stackpole Books, 2006.

Flanders, Judith. *Inside the Victorian Home: A Portrait of Domestic Life in Victorian England*. New York: W. W. Norton & Company, 2003.

Ganguli, Kisari Mohan, translator. *The Mahabharata of Krishna-Dwaipayana Vyasa*. Calcutta: Bharata Press, 1896.

Hand, Wayland D., Anna Casetta, and Sondra B. Thiederman, editors. *Popular Beliefs and Superstitions: A Compendium of American Folklore from the Ohio Collection of Newbell Niles Puckett*. Boston: G. K. Hall, 1981.

Hill, John W., and Doris K. Kolb. *Chemistry for Changing Times*, 9th edition. Upper Saddle River, N.J.: Prentice Hall, 1998, 2001.

Hole, John W., Jr. *Human Anatomy and Physiology*, 5th edition. Dubuque, Iowa: Wm. C. Brown, Publishers, 1978, 1981, 1984, 1987, 1990.

Johnson, Alice A., Janet McKenzie, Hill, Henry HartShorne, Ph.D. *Household Companion: Home Decorations*. Copyright M. L. Dewsnap, 1909.

———. *Household Companion: The Model Cookbook*. M. L. Dewsnap, 1909.

King, Franklin Hiram. *Farmers of Forty Centuries; Organic Farming in China, Korea, and Japan*. New York: Dover Publications, 2004. Originally published: Madison, Wis., 1911.

Kiple, Kenneth F., editor. *The Cambridge World History of Food*. Cambridge, Mass.: Cambridge University Press, 2000.

Kohl, James Vaughn, and Robert T. Francoeur. *The Scent of Eros: Mysteries of Odor in Human Sexuality*. New York: Continuum, 1995.

Leon, Vicki. *Working IX to V*. New York: Walker & Company, 2007.

Levenson, Sam. *Everything but Money*. New York: Simon & Schuster, 1966.

Louv, Richard. *Last Child in the Woods; Saving Our Children from Nature-Deficit Disorder*. Chapel Hill, N.C.: Algonquin Books, 2006.

Mann, Charles C. *1491; New Revelations of the Americas Before Columbus*. New York: Alfred A. Knopf, 2005.

Massey, Lorraine, and Deborah Chiel. *Curly Girl: The Handbook*. New York: Workman Publishing, 2001.

Mertz, Barbara. *Red Land, Black Land: Daily Life in Ancient Egypt*. New York: Peter Bedrick Books, 1990.

Nardi, James B. *Life in the Soil*. Chicago: University of Chicago Press, 2007.

Pond, Caroline M. *The Fats of Life*. Cambridge, Mass.: Cambridge University Press, 1998.

Rombauer, Irma, and Marion Rombauer Becker. *The Joy of Cooking*. Indianapolis, Ind.: The Bobbs-Merrill Company, Inc., 1931, 1936, 1941, 1942, 1943, 1946, 1951, 1952, 1953.

Smith, Huston. *The World's Religions*. San Francisco: Harper, 1958, 1986, 1991.

Stein, Dan. *Dan's Practical Guide to Least Toxic Home Pest Control*. Eugene, Ore.: Hulugosi, 1991.

Tarrow, Susan, translator. *The Written Record of the Voyage of 1524 of Giovanni da Verrazano as recorded in a letter to Francis I, King of France, July 8th, 1524*. New Haven, Conn.: Yale University Press, 1970.

Thich Nhat Hanh. *Old Path White Clouds*. Berkeley, Calif.: Parallax Press, 1991.

Thompson, Daniel V., Jr., translator. *Il Libro dell'Arte—Cennino D'Andrea Cennini. The Craftsman's Handbook (1437)*. New Haven, Conn.: Yale University Press, 1933.

Tyree, Marion Cabell. *Housekeeping in Old Virginia*. Louisville, Ky.: John P. Morton & Company, 1879.

U.S. Department of Agriculture. *Common Weeds of the United States*. New York: Dover Publications, 1971.

Veyne, Paul, editor, and Arthur Goldhammer, translator. *A History of Private Life: Vol. I, From Pagan Rome to Byzantium*. Cambridge, Mass.: The Belknap Press of Harvard University Press, 1987.

Weatherford, Jack. *Indian Givers: How the Indians of the Americas Transformed the World*. New York: Fawcett Columbine, 1988.

Wolverton, B. C. *How to Grow Fresh Air: 50 Houseplants That Purify Your Home or Office*. New York: Penguin Books, 1997.

Zuk, Marlene. *Riddled with Life: Friendly Worms, Ladybug Sex, and the Parasites That Make Us Who We Are*. New York: Harcourt, 2007.

## Lyrics

Geggy Tah. "Special Someone (lyrics)." New York: Luaka Bop, 2007.

## Newspaper Articles

Altman, Lawrence K. "Trial for Vaccine Against H.I.V. Is Canceled." *New York Times,* July 18, 2008.

Bogdanich, Walt. "The Everyman Who Exposed Tainted Toothpaste." *New York Times,* October 1, 2007.

Cole, Carol. "Nail Bacteria Linked to Baby Deaths." Associated Press, March 24, 2000.

Dobson, Roger. "The Oldest Swingers: Sex Games of Stone Age Exposed." *Sunday Times,* April 29, 2007.

Hedin, Jack. "My Forbidden Fruits (and Vegetables)." *New York Times*, March 1, 2008.

Jha, Alok. "Something to Chew Over . . . the Health Benefits of Gum." *Guardian,* March 30, 2006.

Maugh, Thomas H. II, and Marla Cone. "Lead Exposure in Children Linked to Violent Crime." *Los Angeles Times,* May 28, 2008.

Renalls, Candace. "Army Worm Wine." *Duluth News Tribune,* October 31, 2002.

Sail, Stephanie. "Sleep Drugs Found Only Mildly Effective, but Wildly Popular." *New York Times*, October 23, 2007.

Stein, Rob. "FDA Warns Against Giving Cough Medicine to Toddlers." *Washington Post*, August 16, 2007.

## Magazine Articles

Diamond, Jared M. "Evolutionary Biology: Dirty Eating for Healthy Living." *Nature*, 1999.

Gibson, Lydialyle. "The Human Equation." *University of Chicago Magazine*, May/June 2007.

Glines, C. V. "The Cargo Cults." *Airforce Magazine* 74, no. 1, January 1991.

"Jungle Surgery." *Time*, April 28, 1930.

Raffaele, Paul. "In John They Trust." *Smithsonian*, February 2006.

## Government and University Publications and Reports

"Antimicrobial Resistance." Fact sheet, World Health Organization, January 2002.

Brochet, Frédéric: "Chemical Object Representation in the Field of Consciousness." Application for a doctorate from the Faculty of Oenology, General Oenology Laboratory, 351 Cours de la Libération, 33405 Talence Cedex, 2001.

Brooks, Neil, Esq., Julius Krause, Esq., and Edmund Port, Esq. *Crowley's Milk Co. Inc. vs. Brannon, Secretary of Agriculture*. No. 261, Docket 22284. U.S. Court of Appeals Second Circuit, July 23, 1952.

"Cancer Fact Sheet: Cancer of the Kidney and Renal Pelvis 2110–2005." National Cancer Institute.

Donovan, Maryann, Chandra Tiwary, Deborah Axelrod et al. "Medical Hypothesis: Personal care products that contain estrogens or xenoestrogens may increase breast cancer risk." University of Pittsburgh Cancer Institute, 2007.

"Economic Issues with Soybeans." Kansas State University, 2001.

"Environmental Health Network of California '1998 Phthalates Found in Perfume.'" Citizens' Petition filed with the FDA, May 1999.

"EU Reaches Agreement to Impose Ban on Use of Toxics in Cosmetic Products." *Chemical Regulation Reporter*, December 2, 2002.

"Fact Sheet—Hormones in Personal Care Products and the Risk of Breast Cancer in African-American Women." University of Pittsburgh Cancer Institute, February 7, 2006.

"FDA Poisonous Plant Database, March 2006." Revision.

Fellars, Gary, Donald Sparling, and Catherine Puckett. "Research Finds That Breakdown Products of Widely Used Pesticides Are Acutely Lethal to Amphibians." U.S. Department of the Interior, U.S. Geological Survey, May 2007.

Ledoux, Thomas, Ph.D., and Alan Stern, Ph.D. "White Paper Summary on Endocrine Disruption." New Jersey Department of Environmental Protection, Division of Science, Research, and Technology, December 2003.

"National Toxicology Program—Center for the Evaluation of Environmental Health Sciences Expert Panel Report on the Reproductive and Developmental Toxicity of Soy Formula." January 2006.

"National Toxicology Program—Center for the Evaluation of Environmental Health Sciences Expert Panel Report on the Reproductive and Developmental Toxicity of Genistein." April 2006.

"Phthalates and Cosmetic Products." U.S. Food and Drug Administration—Center for Food Safety and Applied Nutrition, March 31, 2005.

"Restless Legs Syndrome Fact Sheet." Revised October 1, 2006. National Institute of Neurological Disorders and Stroke.

Rhodehamel, Jeffry, and Stanley Harmon. "Bacteriological Analytical Manual on-line Bacillus cereus." U.S. Food and Drug Administration, January 2001.

"Spin Master Recalls Aqua Dots—Children Became Unconscious After Swallowing Beads." U.S. Consumer Product Safety Commission, November 7, 2007.

Stamminger, Rainer, Ricarda Badura, Gereon Broil, et al. "A European Comparison of Cleaning Dishes by Hand." Proceedings of EEDAL conference, University of Bonn, Germany, 2003.

"Substances in Cosmetics and Personal Care Products Regulated Under the Food and Drugs Act (F&DA) That Were in Commerce between January 1, 1987, and September 13, 2001." *Health Canada,* 2007

"Tetrodotoxin Poisoning Associated with Eating Puffer Fish Transported from Japan—California, 1996." *Morbidity and Mortality Weekly Report.* Centers for Disease Control and Prevention, May 17, 1996.

Todar, Kenneth. "The Bacterial Flora of Humans." University of Wisconsin–Madison, 2007.

"What are the odds of dying?" National Safety Council, 2003.


### Patent Applications

Novartis AG: "DNA comprising rice anther-specific gene and transgenic plant transformed therewith." EP 1127143 WO 0026389 A20000511.

Scripps Research Institute: Syngenta: "Stress-related genes of plants, transgenic plants containing same, and methods of use." EP 1313867 A2 20030528 WO 02/0166655.

Syngenta: "Abiotic stress responsive polynucleotides and polypeptides." EP 1402042 A2 20040331 WO 2003008540 (170 pages).

Syngenta: "High-protein-phenotype-associated plant genes." WO 03/027249 (163 pages).

Syngenta: "Identification and characterization of phosphate transporter genes." WO 03/000897 (235 pages).

Syngenta: "Identification and characterization of plant genes." EP 1402038 A2 20040331 WO 2003000905 (260 pages).

Syngenta: "Identification and characterization of plant genes." EP 1409696 A2 20030321 WO 2003000904 (323 pages).

Syngenta: "Plant disease resistance genes." EP (European Patent) 1399561 A WO (World Intellectual Property Organization) 03/000906 (299 pages).

Syngenta: "Promoters for plant gene expression." EP 1294914 WO 2001098480 A2 20011227.

Syngenta Aparticipations AG: "Transcription factors of cereals." WO 03/007699 A2 20030130 (125 pages).

Syngenta Participations: "Novel monocotyledonous plant genes and uses thereof." EP 1261715 WO 0166755 A2 20010913.

Syngenta Participations AG: "Oryza sativa nuclea cap binding protein 80." EP 1379659 WO 02081696 A2 20021017.

Syngenta Participations AG: "Nucleic acid molecules from rice encoding proteins for abiotic stress tolerance, enhanced yield, disease resistance and altered nutritional quality and uses thereof." EP 1453950 A2 20040908 WO 2003048319.

Syngenta: "Nucleic acid molecules from rice encoding RARI disease resistance proteins and uses thereof." EP 1539949 WO 2003048339 A2 20030612.

Syngenta: "Nucleic acid molecules from rice controlling abiotic stress tolerance." WO 2005021723 20050310.

Yousef, Ahmed E., Osama O. Ibrahim, and Hyun-jung Chung. "Intracellular proteinacious antimicrobial agents from lactic acid bacteria derived from fermented food samples." U.S. Patent 7112323, September 26, 2006.

## Press Releases

Environmental Working Group. "A benchmark investigation of industrial chemicals, pollutants and pesticides in umbilical cord blood." July 14, 2005. Executive Summary.

————. "Polluted Pets: Chemical exposures and pets' health." April 17, 2008. Executive Summary.

————. "U.S. Health Panel Ignores Science on Food-Packaging Chemical." August 8, 2007.

Hall, Miranda. "University of North Carolina News Release: Soap and water work best in ridding hands of disease viruses." March 11, 2005.

Hansen, Michael, Ph.D.; Jean Halloran; Edward Groth III, Ph.D.; and Lisa Lefferts. Report: "Potential Public Health Impacts of the Use of Recombinant Bovine Somatotropin in Dairy Production." Joint Expert Committee on Food Additives, September 1997.

National Institutes of Health. "Lavender and Tea Tree Oils May Cause Breast Growth in Boys." January 31, 2007. News release.

State University of New York at Buffalo. "New Peptide Derived from Protein in Saliva May Be Promising Antifungal Agent, UB Oral Biologists Find." January 4, 2007. News release.

———. "UB Dental Researchers Find Novel Peptide in Saliva That Kills Broad Range of Fungi and Bacteria." March 5, 2002. News release.

University of California, San Diego. "Warming Climate Plays Large Role in Western U.S. Wildfires, Scripps-Led Study Shows." July 7, 2006. News release.

World Health Organization. "30 percent of diseases in children result from environment." July 27, 2007. News release.

### Scientific Papers

Aas, Johannes, Charles Gessert, and Johan Bakken. "Recurrent *Clostridium difficile* Colitis: Case Series Involving 18 Patients Treated with Donor Stool Administered via a Nasogastric Tube." *Journal of Clinical Infectious Diseases* 36(5), 580–85, 2003.

Alexander, Jan, Diane Benford, et al. "Gossypol as undesirable substance in animal feed; scientific opinion of the panel on contaminants in the food chain." *European Food Safety Authority (EFSA) Journal* 908, 1–55, 2008.

Almond, Christopher, S.D., M.D., M.P.H.; Andrew Shin, M.D.; Elizabeth Fortescue, M.D.; et al. "Hyponatremia Among Runners in the Boston Marathon." *New England Journal of Medicine* 352(15), 1550–56, April 14, 2005.

Anderson, R. C., and J. H. Anderson. "Acute Toxic Effects of Fragrance Products." *Archives of Environmental Health Perspectives* 53(2), 138–46, 1998.

———. "Toxic Effects of Air Freshener Emissions." *Archives of Environmental Health Perspectives* 52(6), 433–41, 1997.

Antonio, M. A., S. E. Hawes, and S. L. Hillier. "The identification of vaginal *Lactobacillus* species and the demographic and microbiologic characteristics of women colonized by these species." *Journal of Infectious Diseases* 180(6), 1950–56, December 1999.

Arulmozhi, D. K., A. Veeranjaneyulu, S. L. Bodhankar, and S. K. Arora. "Effect of *Sapindus trifoliatus* on hyperalgesic in vivo migraine models." *Brazilian Journal of Medical and Biological Research* 38(3), 469–75, March 2005.

———. "Pharmacological investigations of *Sapindus trifoliatus* in various in vitro and in vivo models of inflammation." *Indian Journal of Pharmacology* 37(2), 96–102, April 2005.

Badgley, Catherine, Jeremy Moghtader, Eileen Quintero, et al. "Organic agriculture and the global food supply." *Renewable Agriculture and Food Systems* 22, 86–108, 2007.

Barni, Tullio, Mario Maggi, Guido Fantoni, et al. "Sex Steroids and Odorants Modulate Gonadotropin-Releasing Hormone Secretion in Primary Cultures of

Human Olfactory Cells." *Journal of Clinical Endocrinology & Metabolism* 84(11), 4266–73, 1999.

Bashir, Mohamed Elfatih H., Peter Andersen, Ivan J. Fuss, et al. "An Enteric Helminth Infection Protects Against an Allergic Response to Dietary Antigen." *Journal of Immunology* 169, 3284–92, July 2002.

Beaulieu, Josée, Claude Dupont, and Pierre Lemieux. "Anti-inflammatory potential of a malleable matrix composed of fermented whey proteins and lactic acid bacteria in an atopic dermatitis model." *Journal of Inflammation* 4(6), 2007.

Bellido-Blasco, J., et al. "The effect of alcoholic beverages on the occurrence of a Salmonella food-borne outbreak." *Epidemiology* 13 (2), 228–30, March 2002.

Blackwell, B., S. S. Bloomfield, and C. R. Buncher. "Demonstration to medical students of placebo responses and non-drug factors." *Lancet* 1(7763), 1279–82, June 10, 1972.

Blaser, Martin J. "Who are we? Indigenous microbes and the ecology of human diseases." *European Molecular Biology Organization Reports* 7(10), 956–60, 2006.

Casey, Pat G., Gillian E. Gardiner, Garrett Casey, et al. "A five-strain probiotic combination reduces pathogen shedding and alleviates disease signs in pigs challenged with Salmonella enterica Serovar Typhimurium." *Applied and Environmental Microbiology* 73(6), 1858–63, March 1, 2007.

Cavigelli, Sonia, Jason Yee, and Martha McClintock. "Infant temperament predicts life span in female rats that develop spontaneous tumors." *Hormones and Behavior* 50, 454–62, 2006.

Chorley, Joseph N. "Hyponatraemia: Identification and Evaluation in the Marathon Medical Area." *Sports Medicine* 37(4–5), 451–54, 2007.

Connor, Steve, Michael McCarthy, and Colin Brown. "The end for GM crops: Final British trial confirms threat to wildlife." *Independent*, March 22, 2005.

Davis, E. W. "The ethnobiology of the Haitian zombie." *Journal of Ethnopharmacology* (1), 85–104, November 9, 1983.

Desenclos, J., et al. "The protective effect of alcohol on the occurrence of epidemic oyster-borne Hepatitis A." *Epidemiology* (5), 525–32, 1994.

Eby, George A. "Strong humming for one hour daily to terminate chronic rhinosinusitis in four days: A case report and hypothesis for action by stimulation of endogenous nasal nitric oxide production." *Medical Hypothesis* 66(4), 851–54, 2006.

Edwards, Robert R., Ph.D. "Individual differences in endogenous pain modulation as a risk factor for chronic pain." *Neurology* 65, 437–43, April 5, 2005.

Ernst, E. "Ear candles: a triumph of ignorance over science." *Journal of Laryngology & Otology* 118(1), 1–2, January 2004.

Farnworth, Edward R. "Kefir—a complex probiotic." *Food Science and Technology Bulletin* 2, 1–17, May 2005.

Fisher, Brandy E. "Scents & Sensitivity." *Environmental Health Perspectives* 106(12), November–December 1998.

Fox, Jennifer E., Jay Gulledge, Erika Engelhaupt, et al. "Pesticides reduce symbiotic efficiency of nitrogen-fixing rhizobia and host plants." *Proceedings of the National Academy of Sciences* 104(24), 10282–287, June 4, 2007.

Friedman, M., P. R. Henida, C. E. Levin, and R. E. Mandrell. "Recipes for antimicrobial wine marinades against *Bacillus cereus, Escherichia coli* O157:H7, *Listeria monocytogenes*, and *Salmonella enterica*." *Journal of Food Science* 72(6), M207–13, August 2007.

Geipert, Nadja. "Don't Be Mad." *Monitor on Psychology* 38(1), January 2007.

Gessner, B. D., and M. Beller. "Protective effect of conventional cooking versus use of microwave ovens in an outbreak of salmonellosis." *American Journal of Epidemiology* 139(9), 903–9, May 1, 1994.

Gilberti, Avery N. "Dollars and scents: commercial opportunities in olfaction and taste." *Nature Neuroscience* 5, 1043–45, 2002.

Guarner, Francisco. "Prebiotics in inflammatory bowel diseases." *British Journal of Nutrition* 98, 585–89, 2007.

He, Congrong, Lidia Morawska, and Len Taplin. "Particle Emission Characteristics of Office Printers." *Environmental Science & Technology* 41(17), 6039–45, August 1, 2007.

Henley, Derek, Ph.D.; Natasha Lipson, M.D.; Kenneth Korach, Ph.D.; and Clifford Bloch, M.D. "Prepubertal Gynecomastia Linked to Lavender and Tea Tree Oils." *New England Journal of Medicine* 356(5), 479–85, February 1, 2007.

Hickson, Mary, Aloysius L. D'Souza, Nirmala Muthu, et al. "Use of probiotic *Lactobacillus* preparation to prevent diarrhoea associated with antibiotics: randomised double blind placebo controlled trial." *British Medical Journal* 335, 407–8, June 29, 2007.

Howdeshell, Kembra L., Johnathan Furr, Christy R. Lambright, et al. "Cumulative Effects of dibutyl phthalate and diethylhexyl phthalate on Male Rat Reproductive Tract Development: Altered Fetal Steroid Hormones and Genes." *Toxicological Sciences* 99(1), 190–202, March 30, 2007.

Hunt, John A., Ph.D., FRPharmS. "A short history of soap." *Pharmaceutical Journal*, December 18–25, 1999.

Hunt, Terry. "Rethinking Easter Island's ecological catastrophe." *Journal of Archaeological Science* 34(3), 485–502, 2007.

Ikeda, Takako, Akiyoshi Nishikawa, Takayoshi Imazawa, et al. "Dramatic synergism between excess soybean intake and iodine deficiency on the development of rat thyroid hyperplasia." *Environmental Health Perspectives*, June 2002.

Ingham, John M., and David H. Spain. "Sensual Attachment and Incest Avoidance in Human Evolution and Child Development." *Journal of the Royal Anthropological Institute* 11(4), 677–701, November 8, 2005.

Johnson, V. J., B. Yucesoy, J. S. Reynolds, et al. "Inhalation of toluene diisocyanate vapor induces allergic rhinitis in mice." *Journal of Immunology* 179, 1864–71, July 2007.

Jones, P. A., and D. Takai. "The role of DNA methylation in mammalian epigenetics." *Science* 293(5532), 1068–70, August 10, 2001.

Juhasz-Kaszanyitzky, E. S. Janosi, P. Somogyi, et al. "MRSA transmission between cows and humans." *Emerging Infectious Diseases* 13(4), April 2007.

Keevil, Bill, Ph.D.; James Walker, Ph.D.; and Andrew Maule, Ph.D. "Copper Pipes Kill *E. coli* in Drinking Water." *American Society for Microbiology*, May 22, 2000.

Kogevinas, M. "Human health effects of dioxins: cancer, reproductive and endocrine system effects." *Human Reproduction Update* 7(3), 331–39, 2001.

Lane, T. "Male circumcision reduces risk of both acquiring and transmitting Human Papillomavirus Infection." *International Family Planning Perspectives* 28(3), 179–80, September 2002.

Latch, Douglas E., Jennifer L. Packer, William A. Arnold, and Kristopher McNeill. "Photochemical conversion of triclosan to 2,8-dichlorodibenzo-p-dioxin in aqueous solution." *Journal of Photochemistry and Photobiology* 158(1), 63–66, May 30, 2003.

Lee, M. Y., K. S. Ahn, O. K. Kwon, et al. "Anti-inflammatory and anti-allergic effects of kefir in a mouse asthma model." *Immunobiology* 212(8), 647–54, October 15, 2007.

Liener, Irvin, Ph.D. "Toxic Factors in Edible Legumes and Their Elimination." *American Journal of Clinical Nutrition* 11, 281–98, October 1962.

Lowry, Christopher, Jacob Hollis, Annick De Vries, et al. "Identification of an immune-responsive mesolimbocortical serotonergic system: potential role in regulation of emotional behavior." *Neuroscience* 146(2), 756–72, May 11, 2007.

Lucchelli, P. E., A. D. Cattaneo, and J. Zattoni. "Effect of capsule colour and order of administration of hypnotic treatments." *European Journal of Clinical Pharmacology* 13(2), 153–55, May 17, 1978.

Mastrangelo, Giuseppe, John Grange, Emanuela Fadda, et al. "Lung Cancer Risk: Effect of Dairy Farming and the Consequence of Removing That Occupational Exposure." *American Journal of Epidemiology* 161(11), 1037–46, 2005.

McClintock, Martha K., Susan Bullivant, Suma Jacob, et al. "Human Body Scents: Conscious Perceptions and Biological Effects." *Chemical Senses* 30(1), i135–37, 2005.

McClure, S. M., et al. "Neural Correlates of Behavioral Preference for Culturally Familiar Drinks." *Neuron* 44(2), 379–87, October 14, 2004.

McKinney, P. A., M. Okasha, R. C. Parslow, et al. "Early social mixing and childhood type 1 diabetes mellitus: a case-control study in Yorkshire, U.K." *Diabetic Medicine* 17(3), 236–42, March 2000.

Michon, Richard, and Jean-Charles Chebat. "The Interaction Effect of Background Music and Ambient Scent on the Perception of Service Quality." *Journal of Retailing* 77(2), 273–90, Summer 2001.

Miller, Geoffrey, Joshua Tybur, and Brend Jordan. "Ovulatory cycle effects on tip earnings by lap dancers: economic evidence for human estrus?" *Evolution and Human Behavior* 28(6), 375–81, 2007.

Mitchell, Alyson E., Yun-Jeong Hong, Eunmi Koh, et al. "Ten-Year Comparison of the Influence of Organic and Conventional Crop Management Practices on the Content of Flavonoids in Tomatoes." *Journal of Agricultural and Food Chemistry* 55(15), 6154–59, June 23, 2007.

Montgomery, David R. "Soil erosion and agricultural sustainability." *Sustainability Science* 104(33), 13268–272, August 11, 2007.

Moore, Andrew. "Finding my enemy's enemies." *European Molecular Biology Organization* 5(8), 754–57, August 2004.

Nair, B., and A. R. Elmore. "Final report on the safety assessment of human placental protein, hydrolyzed human placental protein, human placental enzymes, human placental lipids, human umbilical extract, placental protein, hydrolyzed placental protein, placental enzymes, placental lipids, and umbilical extract." *International Journal of Toxicology* 21(1), 81–91, January 2002.

Noakes, Timothy D. "Hydration in the Marathon: Using Thirst to Gauge Safe Fluid Replacement." *Sports Medicine* 37(4–5), 463–66, 2007.

North, K., and J. Golding. "A maternal vegetarian diet in pregnancy is associated with hypospadias." *British Journal of Urology (BJU) International* 85(1), 107–13, January 2000.

Noyce, J. O., H. Michels, and C. W. Keevil. "Inactivation of Influenza A virus on copper versus stainless steel surfaces." *Applied and Environmental Microbiology* 73(8), 2748–50, 2007.

———. "Potential use of copper surfaces to reduce survival of epidemic methicillin-resistant *Staphylococcus aureus* in the healthcare environment." *Journal of Hospital Infections* 63, 289–97, 2006.

O'Brien, M. E., H. Anderson, E. Kaukel, et al. "SRL172 (killed *Mycobacterium vaccae*) in addition to standard chemotherapy improves quality of life without affecting survival, in patients with advanced non-small-cell lung cancer." *Annals of Oncology* 15, 906–14, June 15, 2004.

Pasquina, Paul, M.D.; Kenneth Heilman, M.D.; and Jack Tsao, M.D., D. Phil. "Mirror Therapy for Phantom Limb Pain." *New England Journal of Medicine* 357(21), 2206–7, November 22, 2007.

Patterson, Bruce, Alan Landay, Joan Siegal, et al. "Susceptibility to Human Immunodeficiency Virus-1 Infection of Human Foreskin and Cervical Tissue Grown in Explant Culture." *American Journal of Pathology* 161(3), 867–73, September 2002.

Paul, Ian, M.D., M.Sc.; Jessica Beiler, M.P.H.; Amyee McMonagle, R.N., et al. "Effect of Honey, Dextromethorphan, and No Treatment on Nocturnal Cough and Sleep Quality for Coughing Children and Their Parents." *Archives of Pediatrics & Adolescent Medicine* 161(12), 1140–46, 2007.

Pembrey, M., L. O. Bygren, G. P. Kaati, et al. "Sex-specific, sperm-mediated transgenerational responses in humans." *European Journal of Human Genetics* 14(2), 159–66, February 2006.

Quinn, A. C., A. J. Petros, and P. Vallance. "Nitric oxide: an endogenous gas." *British Journal of Anaesthesia* 74, 443–51, 1995.

Randall, C., H. Randall, F. Dobbs, et al. "Randomized controlled trial of nettle sting for treatment of base-of-thumb pain." *Journal of the Royal Society of Medicine* 93(6), 305–9, June 2000.

Robinson, Thomas, M.D., M.P.H.; Dina Borzekowski, Ed.D.; Donna Matheson, Ph.D.; and Helena Kraemer, Ph.D. "Effects of Fast Food Branding on Young Children's Taste Preferences." *Archives of Pediatrics & Adolescent Medicine* 161(8), 792–97, 2007.

Rodrigues, K. L., L. R. G. Caputo, J. C. T. Carvalho, et al. "Antimicrobial and healing activity of kefir and kefiran extract." *International Journal of Antimicrobial Agents* 25(5), 404–8, May 2005.

Saldana, T. M., O. Basso, J. A. Hoppin, et al. "Pesticide exposure and self-reported gestational diabetes mellitus in the Agricultural Health Study." *Diabetes Care* 30(3), 529–34, July 6, 2007.

San Martín, B., M.V., D.M.V.; J. Kruze, M.V., Ph.D.; M. A. Morales, M.V., Ms.Sc., et al. "Antimicrobial Resistance in Bacteria Isolated from Dairy Herds in Chile." *Journal of Applied Research in Veterinary Medicine* 124(3–4), 319–328, 2002.

Schoen, Edgar, M.D.; Michael Oehrli, M.P.A., C.T.R.; Christopher Colby, Ph.D.; and Geoffrey Machin, M.D. "The Highly Protective Effect of Newborn Circumcision Against Invasive Penile Cancer." *Pediatrics* 105(3), 36, March 2000.

Schweizer, Herbert P. "Triclosan: a widely used biocide and its link to antibiotics." *Microbiology Letters* 202(1), 1–7, June 26, 2001.

Scott, Jordan, M.D.; and Lynda Schneider, M.D. "Factors Associated with the Development of Peanut Allergy in Childhood." *New England Journal of Medicine* 348, 977–85, 2003.

Shiv, Baba, Hilke Plassmann, Antonio Rangel, and John O'Doherty. "Marketing Actions Can Modulate Neural Representations of Experienced Pleasantness." *Proceedings of the National Academy of Sciences* 105(3), 1050–54, January 22, 2008.

Stapleton, Jack, Carolyn Williams, and Jinhua Xiang. "GB Virus Type C: A Beneficial Infection?" *Journal of Clinical Microbiology* 42(9), 3915–19, September 2004.

Steinberg, L. M., F. Odusola, and I. D. Mandel. "Remineralizing potential, antiplaque and antigingivitis effects of xylitol and sorbitol sweetened chewing gum." *Clinical Preventive Dentistry* 14(5), 31–34, September–October 1992.

Summers, R. W., D. E. Elliot, K. Qadir, et al. "Trichuris suis seems to be safe and possibly effective in the treatment of inflammatory bowel disease." *American Journal of Gastroenterology* 98(9), 2034–41, 2003.

Sundar, Krishnan, Qian Liu, Gitty Mousavi, et al. "Hygiene Hypothesis Revisited: Helminthic Infection Prevents Type 1 Diabetes in NOD Mice." *Diabetes* 56(1), A320–21, June 2007.

Tedeschi, Alberto, and Lorena Airaghi. "Is affluence a risk factor for bronchial asthma and type 1 diabetes?" *Pediatric Allergy & Immunology* 17(7), 533–37, November 2006.

Thibodeaux, J. R., and C. Lau. "Exposure to perfluorooctane sulfonate during pregnancy in rat and mouse. I: Maternal and prenatal evaluations." *Toxicological Sciences* 74, 382–92, August 2003.

Venkatesh, Alladi, and Ruby Roy Dholakia. "Households and Technologies: A Socio-Historical Analysis of Two Cultures." Center for Research on Information Technology and Organizations (CRITO), working paper presented at the Association for Consumer Research, International Meeting, Singapore, July 1985.

Walgate, Robert. "Syngenta claims ownership of rice—but will give data away." *Genome Biology Research News*, February 1, 2001.

Wedekind, Claus, Sina Escher, Matthijs Van de Waal, Elisabeth Frei. "The Major Histocompatibility Complex and Perfumers' Descriptions of Human Body Odors." *Evolutionary Psychology* 5(2), 330–43, 2007.

Weidenhamer, Jeffrey, and Michael Clement. "Leaded electronic waste is a possible source material for lead-contaminated jewelery." *Chemosphere* 69(7), 1111–15, April 2007.

Whitten, Patricia L., and Heather B. Patisaul. "Cross-Species and Interassay Comparisons of Phytoestrogen Action." *Environmental Health Perspectives* 109(1), 5–20, March 20, 2001.

Wilks, S. A., H. Michels, and C. W. Keevil. "The survival of *E. coli* O157 on a range of metal surfaces." *International Journal of Food Microbiology* 105, 445–54, 2005.

Williams, L. Keoki, M.D., M.P.H.; Dennis Ownby, M.D.; Mary Maliarik, Ph.D.; and Christine Johnson, Ph.D. "The role of endotoxin and its receptors in allergic disease." *Annals of Allergy, Asthma & Immunology* 94(3), 323–32, March 2005.

Wyart, Claire, Wallace W. Webster, Jonathan H. Chen, et al. "Smelling a Single Component of Male Sweat Alters Levels of Cortisol in Women." *Journal of Neuroscience* 27(6), 1261–65, February 7, 2007.

# INDEX

Aas, Johannes, 201
Aberdeen Organic Hair Treatment, 45
acid rain, 6
acne, 32, 72, 224
adenoviruses, 236
Adlercreutz, Herman, 77
advertising, 25, 107, 186, 194
    fear in, xiii, 2, 12, 15, 135
    odor-related, 17, 19, 21–22
aerosols, 23–24, 40
African Americans, 42, 45–46
aggression, 192–93
agribusiness, 70, 79–87, 93, 125–28
    see also farming
Agriculture Department, U.S.
    (USDA), 64, 89, 96, 97, 128
    crop subsidies by, 63, 65, 67, 77
    food project grants by, 112
Ahn, K. S., 59
AIDS, 234–36, 239
air fresheners, xiii, 17, 22–25, 160
Ak, Nese O., 138
Alexander, S. L., 73
All Detergent Free Clear, 177
Allens Laundry Detergent, 177
allergies, 59, 85, 201
    cleaning and, xiii, 14, 15
Amazon jungle, 242–43

ambergris, 53, 54
Ambien, 185
American Heart Association, 5, 70
American Journal of Clinical Nutrition,
    73, 222
American Lung Association, 226
American Medical Association, 133
amputation, 198–99
Anderson, Lorraine, 72, 73
androgens, 51, 74
animal feed, 88–89, 91, 94–95, 98–99
Antaeus, 60–61
antibiotics, 91, 135, 204
    natural vs. synthetic, 30–31, 59
    see also bacteria, antibiotic-resistant
antifungals, 58, 59
antimicrobials, 56, 58, 111, 136, 150
    dangers of, 49, 132–34, 135, 138
    disposal of, 184
antioxidants, 16
anxiety, 11, 193
apple of love, 51–53
apples, frozen, 116
Applied and Environmental Microbiology,
    98
Aqua Dots, 5
Archer Daniels Midland, 70, 76
Archives of Internal Medicine, 191, 192

Ariely, Dan, 107, 187
art, 107, 128, 241–42
arthritis, 13, 15, 209
    see also joint pain
ASKO, 169
asthma, 24, 42, 59, 101, 220, 226
    cleaning and, xiii, 14
    experimental treatments for, 201,
        208
atherosclerosis, 10, 78
Australia, dairy hormones banned in,
    92
autism, 71–72, 229
autoimmune disorders, xiii, 15, 205,
    206, 207–8
Avon Longitudinal Study of Preg-
    nancy and Childhood, 75
Azerbaijanis, longevity of, 101

bacteria, xiii, 12, 56, 91, 97, 114
    antibiotic-resistant, 30, 133, 134,
        136–37, 138, 201
    beneficial, xii, 49, 58, 132–33, 200,
        201–2; see also probiotics
    in breast milk, 222
    cancer treatment with, 223–24
    foods produced with, 102–4
    in fruits and vegetables, 127
    in hospitals, 135–37
    interactions between humans and,
        102–3, 104
    in kitchens, 135, 139, 149–50
    natural inhibitors of, 30, 58, 204
    removal of, 29, 132, 133–34, 149–50
    in sewage systems, 159
    skin as protected by, 28, 49
    in toilets, 152, 156
    see also microbes; specific bacteria
Baer, William S., 203–4
Bailey, Robert, 235
Bakken, Johan S., 201

baldness, 72
bananas, frozen, 116
barbarians, xii
BASF, 85
bathrooms, 151–66
batteries, 5, 6
Bayer, 85
Beecher, Catharine, 168
beef, 91, 94–95, 96
beer, 103
benzene, 23
benzidines, 175
benzyl acetate, 161
berries, frozen, 116
bile salts, 196
BioCure, 206
Bi-O-Kleen Laundry Detergent, 177
BioMonde, 206
biotechnology, 70, 79–82, 86, 89–92
    see also agribusiness; genetically
        modified (GM) crops
biotherapy, 202–3
birch bark, 55, 143
birds, 215–17
birth control pills, 20, 74
birth defects, 2, 6, 23, 42, 79, 89, 117,
    132, 174, 231, 238
Blaser, Martin, 28
Bloch, Clifford, 50
Block, John R., 67
blood pressure, high, 78, 197
Blum, Robert M., 73
body brushing, 35
body care, 27–61
bone infections, 204
botulism, 114, 223
Boylston, Zabdiel, 228
brain function, 10, 76
    see also memory
brass, antibacterial properties of, 136,
    137

bravery, 9, 10, 26
bread, 142–47
  recipes for, 145–47
breastfeeding, 220–22
breasts, male, 46, 50
Breeze Dryer, 173
brevibacteria, 102
Briggs, Steve, 86
Brochet, Frédéric, 110
Brody, Benjamin, 52
bronze, antibacterial properties of, 137
Buruli ulcer, 30
butane, 23

cabbage, 99–100
cadmium, 163
calcium, 70, 196
Campaign for Safe Cosmetics, 37, 38, 54
Canada, 38, 44, 92
cancer, 41, 42, 58, 99, 117, 174, 201
  bacteria as treatment for, 223–24
  cervical, 233, 236
  colon, 70, 77
  dioxins linked to, 6, 79
  in dogs, 212, 213
  in dry cleaning workers, 181
  penile, 237
  prostate, 70, 72, 76
  testicular, 73
cancer, breast, 46, 50, 100
  soy and, 70, 76, 77
canola, genetically modified, 80–81, 85
Caputo, L. R. G., 58
carbohydrates, 77
carp, 204–5
Casey, Pat G., 98
cats, 213–14
Cavigelli, Sonia A., 9
cavities, 55–57

Center for Food Safety, 81
Centers for Disease Control and
  Prevention, U.S. (CDC), 44, 64,
  126, 130, 135, 190, 222, 223, 230
Central Veterinary Institute, 91
Centre for Applied Microbiology &
  Research (CAMR), 136
Chang, Ellen, 225
Charlie's Soap, 177
Checkoway, Harvey, 224
Cheer, 177
cheese, 102–4
chemicals, 15, 79, 106, 117, 184, 238
  agricultural, 86, 93
  in air fresheners, 23–24, 160
  in cosmetics, 36, 37–38, 39, 40–42
  in drain cleaners, 159
  in fragrances, 161
  in laundry whiteners, 174–76
  lawn, 212, 213, 215, 216–17
  pet exposure to, 212, 213, 215
  in shower curtains, 163
  see also herbicides; pesticides; spe-
    cific chemicals
chickens, 96, 97–98
chicken soup, 116–20
chicle, 55
children, 13, 106, 218–39
  chemical exposure in, 4–5, 212–13
  diseases of, 227, 228–31
  hormone exposure in, 45–46,
    48–49, 51, 54, 73
  hygiene and, 10, 15–16
Children's Hospital of Oklahoma, 135
China, 4, 5–7
  farming in, 69
  garlic production in, 123–25
  infertility in, 88
  traditional medicine in, 187
  traditional waste management in,
    157

Chipotle, 92
chlorhexidine, 56
chlorine, 6, 79, 132, 176
chocolate, health benefits of, 16
cholera, 101
cholesterol, 16, 70, 78, 195–97
    medication for, 190–94
chondroitin sulfate, 120
chromium, 163
Ciabatta Recipe, 147
Cioffi, Eugene, 175
circumcision, 231–38
    AIDS risk lowered by, 233–36
    female, 233
    see also foreskin
civet, 53, 54
Civil War era, health in, 12–13
clay, 30–32, 34
cleaning, xiii, 12, 15, 139, 140, 162,
    241
    see also hygiene
Cliver, Dean O., 138
Clostridium difficile, 134, 137, 201
cloth, cleaning with, 139, 140, 162
clothes drying, 170–73
clothing labels, 181–82
colds, soup as cure for, 120
Coley, William, 223–24
colitis, 201
    ulcerative, xiii, 15, 205, 206
Commonwealth Scientific and In-
    dustrial Research Organization
    (CSIRO), 84, 85
Compleat Cockroach, The (Gordon),
    123
composting, 113, 114, 157, 158, 207
consumerism, xii, xiii, 21–22, 25–26
    environmental impact of, 4, 6–7
    psychology of, 108, 188
    see also shopping
consumer products, 4

safety of, 6–7
Consumer Product Safety Commission
    (CPSC), 4, 5
Consumer Reports, 59
Consumers Union, 181, 197
copper, antibacterial properties of,
    136–37
corn, 63, 77, 83, 85
    see also high-fructose corn syrup
cosmetics, 35–44, 54
    human and animal ingredients in,
        42–44, 45
    modern chemicals in, 39–42
    see also hair dye; lipstick
cotton, 88, 214
    genetically modified, 82–83, 85
cottonseed oil, 85, 88–89
cough syrup, 222–23
coumarin, 174
Country Save Liquid Detergent, 177
cows, 89–92
    cosmetic ingredients from, 44
Creutzfeldt-Jakob disease (CJD),
    44
Crohn's disease, 15, 205, 206, 207
crop subsidies, 63–64, 65–66, 67

daidzein, 72
Dambrine, Étienne, 243
Darwin, Charles, 221
Dawson, Todd, 77
day care, 225
De Cock, Kevin, 235
DeFoliart, Gene, 122
dehydration, 104–6
depression, 193, 202
detergents, 174–80
diabetes, 6, 10, 15, 78, 197, 208
diaminostilbene, 174
diarrhea, 106, 134, 220
diazinon, 216

diet:
    American, 62, 77, 88, 93–94, 95
    vegetarian, 75
digestion, 99, 132, 196, 206
Dimsdale, J. E., 192
dioxins, 6, 79, 132
diphtheria, 230–31
dirt, 12, 28, 29
    health benefits of, xii, 10, 14, 16,
        201–2
dishcloths, 139
dish liquid, 149
dishwashers, 147–48
Djousse, Luc, 195
dogs, 16, 56, 59, 60, 212–13
    air fresheners as harmful to, xiii,
        25
Dow, 85
Downs, Ryan, 100
drains, cleaning, 159–60, 165
Dr. Bronner's Liquid Soap, 33
Dri-Pak Soap Flakes, 178
driving, dangerous, 3, 185
drugs, 184
    statin, 191–94, 196, 197
    see also antiobiotics; medication
dry cleaning, 180–82
DuPont, 76, 85
Durant, Will, 21
dust, 10, 14, 16, 214, 224
Dworkin, Mark, 230
Dyer, Betsey Dexter, 104
dyes, fluorescent, 174–76

ear care, 57–58
ear infections, 220
Eat a Bug Cookbook, The (Gordon),
    123
Eatitworld, 141
Ebell, Mark, 191
Eckel, Robert, 195

ECOS Free and Clear Laundry Deter-
    gent, 177
eczema, 14, 60, 220
Edwin Smith Surgical Papyrus, 231–32
eggs, 16, 96, 97–98, 195
Egyptians, ancient, health and beauty
    practices of, 30, 36, 42, 187,
    231–32
electricity, household use of, 169, 170
electronics, dangerous recycling of, 5–6
Eli Lilly, 92
Elizabeth I, Queen of England, 36
Endangered and Threatened Wildlife
    and Plants List, U.S., 43–44
endocrine system, chemical disrupters
    of, 6, 79, 132, 176
Enriques, Carlos, 138
enterococci, 133
environment, human impact on, 242–43
    see also pollution
Environmental Protection Agency
    (EPA), 42, 79, 116, 181, 214,
    215, 216
Environmental Working Group, 54,
    117, 211, 213
epigenetics, 180
Epstein-Barr virus, 225–26
Erickson, Laura, 216
Ertl, Ronald F., 120
Escherichia coli, 30, 97, 110, 127, 136,
    137
estrogen, 45, 46, 47, 50, 51
    replacement of, 70, 74
EU Directive, 54
Europe, 13, 14, 21–22, 140
European Food Safety Authority, 54
European Union:
    cosmetic ingredients banned in, 38,
        39–40, 42, 44
    dairy hormones banned in, 92
Evangelista, J. C. T., 58

exercise, 189–90
"Experience of the McWilliamses with
　　Membranous Croup" (Twain), 231

fabric softeners, 174
Fair Trade movement, 127
Fargue, Leon-Paul, 102
Farm Act (2002), 63
*Farmers of Forty Centuries: Organic
　　Farming in China, Korea, and
　　Japan* (King), 69, 157
farming, 62, 127, 224
　　chicken, 97–98
　　corporate control of, 80–87
　　dairy, 89–92, 95–96
　　environmental impact of, 93,
　　　125–26, 243
　　organic, 92–93
　　subsidized, 63–64, 65–66
　　urban, 96, 111–13
　　waste management and, 157–58
fat, metabolism of, 78
Fedco Seeds, 87
Federal Bureau of Investigation (FBI),
　　226
Federal Trade Commission (FTC), 90
fertilizers, 69, 93, 126, 156, 243
fingernails, 135
Fish and Wildlife Service, U.S., 215
Fitzpatrick, M. G., 73
flame retardants, 213–14
flatbreads, 144
flavonoids, 70, 71
fleas, 28
Flor, Herta, 199
flouride, 56
Fogel, Robert, 13
food, 62–128
　　cholesterol in, 196
　　cost of, 66, 93, 116, 118, 123–25,
　　　128, 150

genetically modified, 80–82, 84–85
insects as, 122–23
leftover, 115–16, 118
microbes in, 102–3
processed, 68, 77, 88, 94, 111, 128,
　130
waste, 111, 113–14, 115, 116, 144
*see also* farming; *specific foods*
Food and Drug Administration, U.S.
　　(FDA):
　　bovine growth hormones and, 90
　　cosmetic ingredients regulated by,
　　　39, 40, 44
　　cough medicine warnings from, 223
　　inadequacies of, 130–31
　　lead guidelines of, 37, 38
　　medicinal leeches approved by, 202
Food First, 112
food poisoning, 110–11, 114, 130–31,
　　133, 150
food safety, xiii, 101–2, 110–11, 114,
　　126–27, 130–31, 150
food storage, 116, 117, 118, 150
foreskin, 44, 232, 239
forest fires, 153–54
formaldehyde, 23, 41–42
fragrances, 23, 41, 54, 161, 176
　　*see also* perfumes
freegans, 113–14
Freese, Bill, 81
Friedman, Mendel, 110
fruit, 64–66
　　bacteria in, 127
　　frozen, 116
　　salvaging, 114

gamma-hydroxybutyrate (GHB), 5
Gangestad, Steven, 20
Garcia-Houchins, Sylvia, 133
garlic, 123–25
gasoline, 180

gastrointestinal infections, 220
Gause, William C., 208
Gaziano, J. Michael, 195
Geigy Chemical Corporation, 175
genetically modified (GM) crops,
    80–83, 84–87
  environmental effects of, 83–84
genetics, immune system and, 19–20
genistein, 75
Gerba, Charles, 138, 139, 152
German measles, 231
Gessert, Charles E., 201
Giese, Rossman, 30
Gillberg, Christopher, 71
Gillberg, I. Carina, 71
global warming, 153, 154, 243
goiters, 70
golf courses, pesticides on, 216
Golomb, B. A., 191, 192
Gordon, Barney, 83
Gordon, Jeffrey, 200
Gossman, Gail L., 120
gossypol, 88, 89
Grecian Formula, 37
Greeks, ancient, 122, 140
  health and beauty practices of, 36,
    37, 42, 55, 187
GreenEarth Cleaning, 181
Green Housekeeping (Sandbeck), 150,
    160, 182
gum, chewing, 55–56, 57

hair care, 45–48
hair dye, 36–37, 41
hair products, 2, 41, 42
  hormones in, 45–46, 47
Halcion, 185
Hamilton, Marc, 189
handwashing, 29, 131–34, 150
  gels, 133–34
Hangers Cleaners, 181

hay fever, xiii, 207
Health Canada, 57
Healthcare Cost and Utilization Proj-
    ect, 56
heart attacks, 192, 197
  cost of, 56–57
heart disease, 6, 13, 56, 78, 89, 192, 195
  food claims about, 67, 76
  obesity and, 197
  worldwide rates of, 191
heatstroke, 104, 105
Hedin, Jack, 65–66
helminths, 207–8
henna, 36
Hentz, Vincent, 203
herbicides, 80–81, 83–84, 212, 216
herbs, 110–11
herd immunity, 227
hexane, 68
Hibbein, Joseph, 67
high-fructose corn syrup, 77–78
Hippocrates, 197
HIV, 234–36, 239
Hodgkin's disease, 225
home owners' associations, 170–71
honey, as cough treatment, 223
Hong Kong, lead-containing toys
    from, 4
Honolulu Heart Program, 76
Hopi, 57
hormone replacement therapy, 74
hormones, xiii, 23, 41, 54, 196
  in dairy farming, 90–92
  in hair products, 45–46, 47
  male, 72
  sex, 45–46, 48–49, 51, 196
  thyroid, 70, 71–72, 214
  see also estrogen; testosterone
hospitals, hygiene in, 135–37
Household Products Database, 23
Howell, Jimmy Frank, 64

Hudson, Mary Anna, 64
human papillomavirus (HPV), 236–37
humidity, 161, 162, 164
humming, as sinusitis relief, 188–89
hummingbirds, 223
hydroelectric production, 153
hydrogen peroxide, kitchen cleaning
    with, 149–50
hydroquinone, 42
hygiene:
    bathroom, 159–62, 163–65
    hospital, 135–37
    kitchen, 135, 138–39, 149–50
    misconceptions about, 129–30
    personal, 28–29, 33–35
hygiene hypothesis, 14–16
hypochondria, 11, 221
hyponatremia, 104–5
hypospadias, 75
hypothyroidism, feline, 213–14

immune system, 6, 79, 85, 201, 206, 224
    body odor as related to, 19–20
    in children, 225–26, 227
    probiotics as beneficial for, 58, 99
    stress as harmful to, 10
    see also autoimmune disorders
India, 4, 82–83, 93–94
Industrial Revolution, 13
infant formula, 73–74
infertility, 72, 88–89
inflammation, 59, 120, 197
inflammatory bowel disease (IBD),
    205, 206, 207
insects, xii, 122–23
insomnia, 185
insulin resistance, 78
International Rice Genome Sequenc-
    ing Project, 86
iodine, 70
irrigation, 153

Irvine, C. H., 73
isobutane, 23

Jacobs, David, 4
Japan, dairy hormones banned in, 92
Jarvik, Robert, 194
Jews, circumcision of, 232
Johnny's Selected Seeds, 87
Johns Hopkins Medical Institutes, 74,
    234
Johnson, James, 67
joint pain, 120
    see also arthritis
Jordan, Brent D., 18
Joy of Cooking, The (Rombauer), 97, 115

Kaiser Permanente Medical Care
    Program, 237
Kane, T., 192
Kass, Philip H., 138
Kedgeley, Sue, 124
kefir, 58–60, 100–102
Keillor, Garrison, 14
ketchup, as a vegetable, 67
kidneys, 39, 41, 42
kimchi, 99–100
King, F. H., 69, 157
Kirsch, Alan R., 25
kitchens, 129–50
Klietsch, Ronald G., 173
kohl, 36
Kopp, Svenny, 71
Korea, diet in, 100
Kwon, O. K., 59

lactobacilli, 102–3
Lahey, Jim, 145
L'Amande Laundry Soap Flakes,
    176–78
lamb's quarters, 121
land use, 95

laundry, 161, 166–82
    soap, 168, 174, 176
    whiteners, 174–76, 177
lavender, 49, 50
Lazy Bread for Napkins, 145–47
lead, 4–5, 6
    in candles, 215
    in cosmetics, 36, 37–38
    in shower curtains, 163
leeches, 202–3, 206
legumes, toxins produced by, 68–69
Lehman's, 173
leprosy, 30
leukemia, 6, 212, 213, 224
Levine, James, 190
Li, Su-Ting, 46
lice, 28
life expectancy, xii, 12
linens, bath, 161–62, 165
Lipitor, 194
lipstick, 37–38
listeria, 97, 110
liver, 39, 41, 42, 54, 89
    cholesterol synthesis in, 196
    PFOSs as damaging to, 174
L'Oréal, 38
Lowry, Christopher, 201
Lund, Trent, 72
lung disease, 56
luteinizing hormone, 45
Lux Soap Flakes, 178
lymphoma, 212, 224
Lynda (author's friend), 209

McClintock, Martha K., 9, 18, 19
McKay, Andrew, 81
Madsen, Kreesten M., 229
Maggie's Pure Land, 180
maggots, 203–4, 206, 240
Maimonides, 120
malaria, 13

marathoners, 104, 105
marketing, 108
    see also advertising; consumerism
mastic, 55
Mastrangelo, Giuseppe, 224
matches, as air fresheners, 160, 165
Mather, Cotton, 228
Matthews, Donald, 64
Mayans, 55
Mayo Clinic, 189
measles, 13, 228–29
    German, 231
Medical University Children's Hospital, 101
medication, 39, 185–87
    anticholesterol, 190–94, 196, 197
    children's, 222–23
    disposal of, 184
    natural, 200–209
    see also drugs
meditation, 188–89
Mehta, Pradeep S., 93
memory, 5
    gum-chewing as beneficial to, 55
    toxin exposure and, 180
meningitis, bacterial, 220
Mennella, Julie, 20
menopause, 70, 74, 76
menstrual cycle:
    pheromone release in, 18
    soy milk and, 70
Merck, 235
mercury, 163, 229
    in cosmetics, 36, 38–39, 40
    in pets, 212
    in vaccines, 229
metabolic syndrome, 78
metabolism, 70, 189, 190, 196
methicillin-resistant Staphylococcus aureus (MRSA), 30, 91, 133, 136, 137

Mexico, farming in, 63
Microban, 138
microbes, 102–3
    beneficial, 16, 131, 200–202
    skin-dwelling, 27–28, 131, 134, 200
    *see also* bacteria
microfiber, washing with, 32
Mielke, Howard, 37
migrant workers, 126
mildew, in bathrooms, 161, 162, 164
milk, 89–92
    fermented, 58, 98, 100–101
    soy, 68–69
Miller, Geoffrey, 18
mirror therapy, 199
Moe, Christine, 133, 134
mold, 114, 161, 164
mononucleosis, 225–26
Monsanto, 70, 79–83, 84, 85, 90, 91, 92
Montague, Read, 106
mortality, cholesterol and, 191–92
Mountain Rose Herbs, 31
Mousavi, Gitty, 208
Muhammed, K. K., 31
Muir, Cameron, 51
musk, 53, 54
Muslims, circumcision of, 232
*Mycobacterium tuberculosis*, 133, 138
*Mycobacterium ulcerans*, 30
*Mycobacterium vaccae*, 201–2

nail polish, solvents in, 5
napkins, 140–41
National Audubon Society, 215
National Institutes of Health (NIH), 11, 23, 185, 186, 187, 235
National School Lunch Program, 66
Native Americans, 13–14, 55, 242
Natural Medicine Research Center, 101

Natural Resources Defense Council, 23
Nature with Love, 180
Neaton, James, 192
Neem Resource, 180
nervous system, 38, 39, 44
    chemicals interfering with, 23, 42
    cholesterol as integral to, 196
Newman, Susie, 144
*New York Times*, 65, 83, 143, 145
New Zealand, 92
nitric oxide, production of, 188, 189
No Knead Bread, 143, 145
nonexercise activity thermogenesis (NEAT), 190
nonstick cookware, 117, 212, 215
noroviruses, 133–34
North American Free Trade Agreement (NAFTA), 63

obesity, 77–78, 190, 197, 221–22
    childhood, 226, 227
O'Brian, Mary, 201
odors, 17–21, 102
    aphrodisiac effects of, 25
    body, 19, 21, 51–53
    household, 160–61
olive oil, 34–35, 48
omega-3 fatty acids, 95
*101 Ways to Help Birds* (Erickson), 216
Onesimus, 228
*Organic Housekeeping* (Sandbeck), 150, 160, 182, 241
Osmond, T. E., 232
osteoporosis, 76
Oughton, Michael, 134
Ovid, 42, 61

pain:
    in children, 219–20
    chronic, 197–98, 199–200

male sensitivity to, 237–38
phantom, 198–99
paint, 5, 37, 41
parasites, 28
intestinal, 10, 15, 205–8
Park, Kun-Young, 99
patents, agricultural, 81–82, 86–87
Paul, Ian M., 223
peas, genetically modified, 84–85
perchloroethylene, 180–81
Perfecto, Ivette, 92, 93
perfluorinated (PFOS) products, 174
perfluorochemicals, 212
perfumes, 53–54, 161
see also fragrances
pertussis, 230
Pesticide Action Network North
America, 88
pesticides, 5, 49, 84, 85, 88, 126, 127
birds as poisoned by, 215–16
childhood cancers linked to,
212–13
Peters, Chris, 95
petroleum, petroleum products, 25, 26,
68, 93, 126, 164, 176, 214
pets, xiii, 14, 211–17
food for, 130
see also birds; cats; dogs
pharmaceutical industry, 184–87, 194,
197, 223
pheromones, 18–19, 53
phimosis, 232, 238
phosphates, 176
phosphorus, 70, 155, 196
phthalates, 23, 41, 54, 132, 163
Physicians' Health Study, 195
phytoestrogens, 70, 71, 72–74, 75,
76–77
pigs, 93, 96, 98–99
pinworms, 207
placebos, 187–88, 222

placenta, 45, 47
Planet Ultra, 177
plants, as air fresheners, 160, 165
plastics, 6, 137, 138, 141
Pliny the Elder, 42, 122
pneumonia, 133
pollution, 3–7, 31, 38, 54, 141
agricultural, 93, 125–26
antimicrobials as cause of, 132
water, xiii, 132, 153, 155–56, 175,
176, 184
polybrominated diphenyl ethers (PB-
DEs), 213–14
polyurethane foam, 214
potatoes, 117, 119
pregnancy, 20, 56
thyroid hormone levels in, 71–72
preservatives, mercury-based, 39
prions, 44
probiotics, 58, 98–102, 222
see also bacteria, beneficial
progesterone, 51, 74
propane, 23
propionibacteria, 102
prostaglandins, 45
protein, insects as source of, 122
Pseudomonas aeruginosa, 138
Pseudomonas stutzeri, 30
psoriasis, 204–5
puberty, premature, 45–46, 48–49, 73
purslane, 121

Ramachandran, Vilayanus S., 198–99
Raverat, Gwen, 221
recombinant Bovine Growth Hormone (RGBH), 90–92
recycling, 5–6
red clover, 74
Reigstad, Ray, 109
Rennard, Barbara O., 120
Rennard, Stephen I., 120

reproductive problems, 6, 23, 38, 41, 73, 75, 79, 89, 132
reproductive system, male, 75
Requip, 186–87
respiratory problems, 42, 220, 224
restless leg syndrome, 186–87
Restoril, 185
rheumatic fever, 13
risk taking, 226, 240–43
Robbins, Richard A., 120
Román, Gustavo C., 71
Romans, ancient, 122, 140, 167, 243
    health and beauty practices of, 34, 37, 38, 42–43, 187, 209
Rombauer, Irma, 97
Roundup Ready crops, 80–81, 82, 83–84
rubella, 231
Russell, Bertrand, 171

saliva, 51, 55, 59
    antimicrobial properties of, 60
salmonella, 97, 98–99, 101, 133, 138
Salmonella enterica, 110
Salmonella typhimurium, 30, 127
salt, in soup, 119
Schmeiser, Percy, 80–81, 87
Schmucker, Douglas Lees, 101
Schneedorf, J. M., 58
Schneider, Jill E., 73
Scholey, Andrew, 55
school lunches, 66–67
Schwab, Charles, 64
Schwarzenegger, Arnold, 153
Schweizer, Herbert P., 138
Scotchgard, 173–74
Scott Paper Company, 141
Scripps Institution of Oceanography, 153
Sea of Galilee, 153
sea turtles, 43–44

Sea World, 43
September 11, 2001, terrorist attacks of, xii
severe acute respiratory syndrome (SARS), 3, 100
sex, testosterone's role in, 51
sexually transmitted diseases, 233–36
Shakespeare, William, 4
Sharma, A. K., 89
shopping, xii, 7–9
shower curtains, 163
sinusitis, 188–89
skin, 39, 41–44, 51, 198, 202
    disorders of, 41, 60, 204–5
    dry, olive oil treatment for, 34–35
    function of, 27–28
    microbes in, 28, 49, 102, 131, 132, 134, 200
    toxins absorbed through, 35–36, 41, 42, 54
smallpox, 228
smells, see odors
soap, 28, 30, 131–33, 134, 163–64
    castile, 33, 164, 165
    laundry, 168, 174, 176
soap nuts, 178–80
social mores, 16–17, 111, 122
soft drinks, 77–78, 106–7
solvents, 5, 41, 68, 180–81
soup, 115, 117–20, 121
South Korea, garlic tariffs in, 124–25
soy, soy products, 63, 67–77
    autism and, 71–72
    genetically modified, 83–84, 85
    health effects of, 67, 70, 72, 76–77
    in infant formula, 73–74
    phytoestrogens in, 70, 71, 72–74, 75, 76–77
    prenatal effects of, 74–75
sperm, 6, 72–73, 75
spices, 110–11

sponges, bacteria in, 139
spongiform encephalopathy, 44
sports drinks, 104, 105, 107–8
Stanford, John, 224
Stanley, Arthur, 158
staphylococcus, 58, 91
*Staphylococcus aureus*, 30, 91, 222
statin drugs, 191–94, 196, 197
steel, stainless, bacteria as thriving on, 136, 137
Sternberg, Wendy, 237
steroid hormones, 48–49, 196
stinging nettle, 121, 209
Stockman, David, 67
streptococcus, 30
*Streptococcus mutans*, 56
*Streptococcus pneumoniae*, 133
stress, chronic, 10
stroke, 5, 56, 197
Suarez, Edward, 193
sugar, 77
Sundar, Krishnan, 208
Surf Powder, 177
Swanson, Jamie, 73
sweat, 19, 20, 28, 104, 105
    sex hormones in, 51
Swetnam, Thomas, 154
Syngenta, 85, 86

Tah, Geggy, 51
tar, black, 55
Taylor, Susan, 171
tea tree, 49, 50
*terra preta do Indio*, 242–43
testosterone, 6, 45, 48, 51, 75
thimerosal, 229
Thoreux, Karine, 101
3M, 173
thyroid, 70, 71–72, 89, 214
Tiwary, Chandra, 46
tofu, 69, 76

toilet paper, 161, 165
toilets, 152, 154–58
    cleaning of, 165
tooth care, 55–57
tortillas, 144
toxins, genetic effects of, 180
toys, lead in, 4, 5
trenchers, 142
triclosan, 132, 138
Tschöp, Matthias, 77
tuberculosis, 13, 30, 133, 201
Twain, Mark, 1, 231
Tybur, Joshua M., 18
typhoid, 13

United Farm Workers Union, 127
United Nations, 86, 94
Urban Clothes Lines, 173
urinals, waterless, 156–57
urinary problems, 220, 236, 238
urine:
    as ancient laundry detergent, 167
    disposal of, 154–57
*USA Today*, 223

vaccinations, 227–31
vaccines, 12, 229
    HIV, 235–36
Vasan, Ramachandran, 78
vegetables, 64–67
    bacteria in, 126–27
    salvaging of, 114
    in school lunches, 66–67
    for soup, 117
Velasquez-Pereira, J., 89
Vermont Country Store, 173
Verrazano, Giovanni da, 14
Veterans Affairs Medical Center, 204
Vick's Vapo Rub, 59
Vine, Donna, 78

vinegar:
  bathroom cleaning with, 164–65
  kitchen cleaning with, 149–50
  skin cleansing with, 32
vinyl, 41, 163
virtual reality therapy, 199
viruses, 12, 14
  in children, 225–26
  handwashing gels and, 133–34
  kefir as protection from, 58
vitamin D, 196
volatile organic compounds (VOCs),
    163

Wal-Mart, 8, 92
Wansink, Brian, 108
Ward, Mary H., 212, 213
WashEZE, 177
washing machines, 168–69
*Washington Post*, 64, 67
waste, 17
  food, 111, 113–14, 115, 116, 144
  human, 154–58
water:
  conservation of, 32
  consumption of, 104–6, 107
  hard, 164
  household use of, 148, 155–56, 169
  supplies of, 153, 154
Waterless No-Flush, 157
water pollution, xiii, 132, 153, 155–56,
    175, 176, 184

Wedekind, Claus, 19, 20
Wedgwood, Emma, 221
Weidenhamer, Jeffrey, 6
Weinstock, Joel, 205
West Nile virus, 3
wheat, subsidized, 63
whipworms, 206–7
White, Lon, 76
whooping cough, 230
wine, 108, 109–11
Wong, Ming H., 6
wood, antibacterial properties of, 138
Woolite, 177
World Bank, 4
Worldcentric, 141
World Health Organization, 3, 6, 228,
    229
wounds, leeches and maggots for,
    202–4
Wysocki, Charles, 20

xylitol, 55–56

yeast, 103
yogurt, 102

Zacharias, J. F., 203
Zahm, Sheila Hoar, 212, 213
Zdravic, F., 202
ZeroFlush, 157